DATE			

© THE BAKER & TAYLOR CO.

THE
LIFE
YOU
SAVE

THE
LIFE
YOU
SAVE

A guide to getting the best possible care from doctors, hospitals, and nursing homes

by LEWIS MILLER

WILLIAM MORROW AND COMPANY, INC.
NEW YORK   1979

Library of Congress Catalog Card Number 78-1728

ISBN 0-688-03461-6

CARL WEISS   BOOK DESIGN

Printed in the United States of America.

First Edition

1   2   3   4   5   6   7   8   9   10

To Jean, for her patient care

PREFACE

LEW MILLER HAS SPENT MOST OF HIS PROFESSIONAL LIFE getting the latest information out of doctors who had some special expertise and disseminating it to their colleagues. He concentrated on helping doctors in a non-medical fashion when he served as editor of *Medical Economics,* during which era it was my privilege to serve as a contributing editor under Lew's guidance and to get to know Lew personally.

When he left *Medical Economics* to found *Patient Care* magazine I was saddened not only because I had enjoyed working with Lew but because I honestly did not believe it would be possible for a medical magazine to deal with the broad spectrum of medical practice that Lew envisioned as the target of *Patient Care.*

I was wrong. Within a year Lew was publishing a magazine that covered a vast array of medical topics, always in an interesting, informative style. Lew obviously had a gift for eliciting from physicians the most pertinent, up-to-date medical information available and he had a flair for presenting it in a readable, useful format. *Patient Care* deservedly became a great success.

Now Lew has used his same skills to do for the patient what he did for physicians. His broad experience in all the fields of medicine, the knowledge he has acquired which enables him to find the best possible sources of information, and his ability to present all this information in a most readable style makes *The Life You Save* a truly valuable book.

I unhesitatingly predict it will do more to help patients deal wisely and successfully with every facet of our complex medical system than any book, by doctor or lay person, previously written. I recommend it with great enthusiasm.

WILLIAM A. NOLEN, M.D.

ACKNOWLEDGMENTS

THIS BOOK HAS BEEN IN THE MAKING FOR MORE THAN TEN years. I finished the manuscript thanks only to the persistent encouragement of my wife, Jean, my son, David, my daughter, Kathy, and my longtime friend and editor, Howard Cady. Now I can look all four in the eye again, and I feel a more conscientious, if not healthier, person for having summed up my years of health-care experience in the chapters that follow.

I owe debts of gratitude to two erstwhile editorial colleagues who helped me research and shape some of the chapters: Gene Balliett, now a professional management consultant, and Don Lamb Witty, now a portrait artist. Also to a distinguished group of professional reviewers who sought to straighten out my biases and to correct my medical and statistical statements:

Lynn Carmichael, M.D., professor and chairman, Department of Family Medicine, University of Miami School of Medicine, Miami, Florida;

Donald Carner, executive vice president, Memorial Hospital, Long Beach, California;

William C. Felch, M.D., internist of Rye, New York, former president of the American Society of Internal Medicine;

Edward A. Felder, M.D., of Darien, Connecticut, a longtime friend and associate (and our family doctor before he gave up practice);

Thomas R. Godkins, P.A., director of the Physician's Associate Program, University of Oklahoma Health Sciences Center, Oklahoma City;

C. Stratton Hill, Jr., M.D., endocrinologist and associate director (clinics), M. D. Anderson Hospital and Tumor Institute, Houston, Texas;

Leslie B. Huffman, M.D., family physician of Maumee,

Ohio, former president of the American Academy of Family Physicians;

Harold B. Kaiser, M.D., internist and allergist, Minneapolis, Minnesota;

Sam A. Nixon, M.D., family physician and director, Division of Continuing Education, University of Texas Health Sciences Center, Houston;

Leonard Rubin, M.D., internist and director of education, Kaiser Permanente Clinics, Oakland, California;

William E. Ryan, senior executive vice president, Blue Cross–Blue Shield, Chicago;

Steven Sieverts, vice president, New York Blue Cross, New York City;

Anne R. Somers, professor of family and community medicine, Rutgers University School of Medicine, Piscataway, New Jersey, and a well-known author on the health-care system;

Leon E. Warshaw, M.D., vice president and corporate medical director, Equitable Life Assurance Society of the U.S., New York City;

J. Jerome Wildgen, M.D., family physician, Kalispell, Montana, and past president, American Academy of Family Physicians.

Thanks too to William A. Nolen, M.D., the famous surgeon-author (or author-surgeon now) of Litchfield, Minnesota, whom I encouraged in the embryonic days of his writing career and who now has written the preface for this book.

The credit for the valuable ideas and information in this book goes not only to these dedicated people but also to the hundreds of physicians, other health professionals, and patients who have shared their experiences with me over the past eighteen years. But I take the responsibility for the factual accuracy of the content and for the opinions expressed herein.

By the way, I have liberally mixed fact and fiction in my efforts to describe medical-care problems anecdotally. The experiences are true but have been disguised to protect people and institutions. In general, I have identified correctly physicians, patients, or others from whom I have quoted directly.

My good friend August A. Fink, Jr., Ph.D., with whom I founded *Patient Care* magazine, was kind enough to allow me to quote and adapt much material from that popular medical journal. Three secretaries, Susan Turkington, Rina Plotkin, and Karen Lehn, have made sense of my discursive dictation and rambling scrawls.

Since my consciousness was raised during the decade in which I wrote this book, I hope you will pardon any inappropriate gender references that slipped through. So whenever you see "he," "him," or "his," please also read "she," "her," or "hers."

If you, the reader, find one or two ideas you can use in future experiences with doctors, hospitals, or nursing homes, I will feel my efforts have been rewarded.

LEWIS MILLER

Darien, Connecticut
January, 1979

CONTENTS

PREFACE   7

ACKNOWLEDGMENTS   8

CHAPTER 1 : *THE LIFE YOU SAVE*

It's your life, not the doctor's . . . Doctors are human too . . . Information should be fully imparted . . . Your expectations should be realistic . . . Costs are high, so make the most of what's available . . . You have the right to know and to say no.   *21*

CHAPTER 2 : *CHOOSING A DOCTOR*

The most common errors . . . Choices for a primary physician . . . When an internist is better than a family physician and vice versa . . . Individual, partnership, or group practice . . . Nine ways to find the doctor you want.   *28*

CHAPTER 3 : *WHICH SPECIALIST FOR YOU?*

When to seek a specialist yourself . . . When to ask your family doctor . . . How to evaluate credentials, including certification . . . Precautions to observe . . . Description of major specialties.   *36*

CHAPTER 4 : *THOSE NON-M.D. DOCTORS*

Who they are . . . When to use osteopaths, psychologists, podiatrists, optometrists . . . What about chiropractors?   *46*

12 /

CHAPTER 5 : *SHOULD YOU SEE A
"PHYSICIAN EXTENDER"?*

Growing numbers of physicians' assistants and nurse
practitioners . . . Their value in certain practices and in
rural areas . . . Cautions on independent nurse practitioners.   *51*

CHAPTER 6 : *HOW OFTEN DO YOU NEED
A CHECKUP?*

Are checkups a waste of time? . . . Value of early detection of disease . . . What doctors say about checkups
. . . Health Hazard Appraisal . . . Frequency of checkups by age . . . What should be included in childhood,
middle years, old age . . . Where to have a checkup . . .
Costs . . . Checklists of tests.   *55*

CHAPTER 7 : *WHICH SIGNS AND SYMPTOMS
REQUIRE A DOCTOR?*

Difficulty of telling what is serious and what isn't . . .
Emergencies that require immediate action . . . Guidelines for when to call the doctor . . . Doctors have problems, too . . . Checklist of serious symptoms.   *70*

CHAPTER 8 : *WHAT TO TELL THE DOCTOR*

Importance of the history . . . Clues to diagnosis . . .
Dangers of withholding information . . . Differing types
of medical histories and their value.   *82*

CHAPTER 9 : *WHAT TO ASK YOUR DOCTOR—
IN THE OFFICE*

Problems in communications . . . Value of open exchange . . . Patient complaints . . . Guidelines to getting
the information you need . . . Ask for details on shots,
drugs, tests, therapy . . . Get it in writing . . . Find out
the prognosis . . . You have a right to know.   *91*

CHAPTER 10 : *WHAT TO ASK ABOUT*
PERSONAL PROBLEMS

The hidden questions . . . How to overcome embarrassment or fear in asking . . . Specific clues on introducing topics of sex, marital conflict, mental illness, alcoholism . . . Checklist for women. *100*

CHAPTER 11 : *"THEY SAY IT'S CANCER"*

Value of second opinion . . . Where to find experts . . . Types of treatment . . . Pursuit of untried therapies . . . Quality of life a factor . . . Growth of home care. *107*

CHAPTER 12 : *A POCKET HEALTH RECORD*
Memory can fail you and your doctor . . . The problems of transferring medical information . . . How to keep your personal record up to date to avoid problems . . . Your own Personal Health Profile. *112*

CHAPTER 13 : *HOW MUCH ATTENTION*
SHOULD YOU EXPECT FROM
YOUR DOCTOR?

Time is vital to you and the doctor . . . Getting an appointment . . . Waiting time . . . Treatment time . . . Advice by phone . . . House calls . . . If the doctor isn't available . . . Hospital visits. *118*

CHAPTER 14 : *HOW CAN YOU TELL IF YOUR*
DOCTOR IS GIVING YOU GOOD
CARE?

Difficulty of judging . . . Outcome or process measurements . . . What to look for . . . Are you getting better? . . . Differences among doctors' own evaluations. *130*

CHAPTER 15 : *WHEN SHOULD YOU GET*
ANOTHER DOCTOR'S OPINION?

You should make the decision . . . Five situations in which to get a second opinion . . . How to pick a consultant, with your doctor's help. *137*

14 /

CHAPTER 16 : *WHAT TO DO IF YOU'RE*
DISSATISFIED WITH YOUR
DOCTOR

Problem physicians and problem patients . . . When to
talk to your doctor about your complaints . . . If personality is the problem . . . Incompetence or malpractice? . . . Grounds for a lawsuit . . . Informed consent . . .
Reasonable care . . . Good supervision . . . Abandonment . . . How to handle grievances . . . When to get a
lawyer. *143*

CHAPTER 17 : *WHEN AND WHY TO GO*
INTO THE HOSPITAL

A place to die or a place to revive? . . . New technologies available . . . Previous indications changing . . .
Use of outpatient surgery . . . Preventing hospitalization . . . Questions to ask the doctor. *153*

CHAPTER 18 : *WHAT TO ASK YOUR DOCTOR—*
IN THE HOSPITAL

Don't wait to ask . . . Don't be intimidated by specialists,
residents, and nurses . . . Fundamental rights of the
patient . . . Guidelines on what to ask about treatment,
risks, second opinions, recovery time . . . Put it in
writing. *157*

CHAPTER 19 : *HOW TO CHOOSE A HOSPITAL*

Where your doctor has privileges . . . Accreditation . . .
General or special services . . . Pros and cons of teaching hospitals . . . Is bigger better? . . . Nonprofit or
investor-owned? . . . Doctors' privileges . . . Warning
signs. *164*

CHAPTER 20 : *HOW TO EVALUATE HOSPITAL CARE*

Compassion plus care . . . Who monitors quality of care? . . . Coordination of care . . . Primary nursing . . . Patient representatives . . . Nursing care . . . Food . . . Buildings . . . Financial status . . . Patient's Bill of Rights. *171*

CHAPTER 21 : *WHICH TYPE OF LONG-TERM CARE IS BEST?*

The dilemma of the aging ill . . . Role of relatives . . . Extended-care facilities . . . Nursing-care facilities . . . Residential care . . . Foster homes . . . Home health care . . . Day-care centers . . . How to decide which to choose for patient and family. *181*

CHAPTER 22 : *WHAT TO LOOK FOR IN A NURSING HOME*

Are good food and kindness enough? . . . Look at the patient's needs . . . Check services offered . . . The "little things" . . . Physical plant . . . Livable, not institutional . . . Licensing . . . Costs . . . A personal visit . . . Checklist for evaluation. *189*

CHAPTER 23 : *WHAT YOU NEED TO KNOW ABOUT HEALTH INSURANCE*

Beware variations in benefits and coverages . . . How much coverage is enough? . . . A "best buy" type of policy . . . Look at the exclusions . . . What to look for in your own coverage . . . Hospital, surgery, office care, and other benefit options . . . How long do benefits last? . . . Service vs. indemnity benefits . . . Major medical plans . . . Cautions on policy restrictions . . . Health Maintenance Organizations . . . How to improve your group or individual coverage . . . Guidelines for family coverage. *200*

CHAPTER 24 : *TIPS ON MEDICARE AND MEDICAID COVERAGE*

40 million covered by government programs . . . Confusing regulations . . . Differences between the two plans . . . Who's eligible . . . Benefits and deductibles . . . Doctor's charges . . . What to ask the doctor . . . Finding a Medicare or Medicaid doctor . . . Disputed claims . . . Where to get more help.   *214*

CHAPTER 25 : *HOW CAN YOU TELL IF THE DOCTOR'S BILL IS FAIR?*

$50 or $1 for an office visit? . . . Wide ranges by specialty and by region . . . Effects of health insurance on fees for service . . . Rapid rise in charges . . . How doctors set fees . . . Should specialists get more? . . . Surgical vs. medical fees . . . Lab and X-ray charges . . . Relative-value scales . . . Discuss fees in advance . . . Compare with others in region, but not with Medicare.   *221*

CHAPTER 26 : *WHAT YOU SHOULD KNOW ABOUT HOSPITAL AND NURSING-HOME CHARGES*

Wide variation by type of hospital and location . . . Rapid increase in service costs, including labor . . . New technology . . . Insurers pay different rates . . . Physicians not well informed . . . Check your bill . . . Nursing-home charges.   *230*

CHAPTER 27 : *WHAT TO DO IF YOU'RE DISSATISFIED ABOUT A BILL*

Preventing the problem . . . Getting an explanation . . . Appealing to the medical society . . . When to see a lawyer . . . Tips on hospital-bill complaints.   *237*

CHAPTER 28 : *WHAT TO DO ABOUT RISING HEALTH-CARE COSTS*

Waste by doctors and hospital personnel . . . Cooperate with your doctor . . . Shorten your hospital stay . . . 10 ways to monitor hospital costs . . . How to hold down nursing-home costs . . . 10 steps to cut down on doctor bills . . . Change your life-style . . . Help avoid costly duplication. *241*

CHAPTER 29 : *CAN YOU REALLY MEASURE QUALITY OF MEDICAL CARE?*

The experts can't define it . . . Looking at what's done . . . The results of care . . . The use of resources . . . Patient satisfaction . . . What states, medical societies, and hospitals are doing . . . How the government monitors quality . . . Maintaining quality at lower cost . . . The United States ahead of other countries. *250*

APPENDIX :
Health History Questionnaire *259*

INDEX *273*

THE
LIFE
YOU
SAVE

1

THE LIFE YOU SAVE

THIS IS A BOOK ABOUT THE MEDICAL-CARE SYSTEM AND WAYS you can make better use of it with all its strengths and weaknesses, to help you make the most of your life and health. It is based on the lessons I have learned about doctors over the past twenty years—lessons that have made me neither more cynical about them nor more protective of them. Rather, I have found *for myself* a new understanding of my life and my health in relation to the medical-care system. My life is the only one I have. It is up to *me* to protect it and to keep it healthy. My life and my health are *not* the doctor's responsibility, unless and until I specifically delegate some of that responsibility to him. This is a new concept for many patients and their doctors.

Over the years, some doctors have been willing to play God, and patients have been even more willing to allow them to play that role, particularly when the problem appears to be serious. We should be through with those days. What can be more condescending than having an MDeity pat a young woman on the head as he leaves her half-draped on the examining-room table, saying, "Don't you worry. You're going to be all right, little lady!" But it is taking us a long time to get rid of the images and relationships that have been created—a long time on the part of both doctors and patients. On both sides, there needs to be an understanding that each of us is responsible for his or her own health and health care, and that the doctor, the hospital, and the rest of the medical-care system are available resources to use.

I came to this realization slowly, and only by getting to know a great deal about the medical-care system and what it can, and can't, do for people. My close day-to-day association with practicing physicians started in 1960 when I became executive editor of *Medical Economics,* a business and professional magazine for doctors, and intensified in 1966 when I founded and served as editor-in-chief of *Patient Care,* a practical clinical journal for primary physicians. To be a good magazine editor means you must know your readers and their needs for information. So I set out to learn as much about practicing physicians as I could.

To do this, I traveled the medical highways of the United States and other countries. I sat in countless waiting rooms and talked to patients. I watched hundreds of physicians work in their examining rooms. I made house calls and hospital rounds with them. I visited in their living rooms and at their kitchen tables and listened to their joys and sorrows, their gripes and triumphs, as fellow human beings.

I recall making rounds in a nursing home with an old friend, a sixty-year-old family doctor I'll call Ted Klein. As we visited room after room, Dr. Klein bent over each elderly patient—whether they needed his medical services or not—to pass along a few words of hope, encouragement, or personal flattery ("You really look beautiful today, Mrs. Smith"). He touched a forehead or held a gnarled, arthritic hand when the occasion called for it, he moved a glass of water within reach of a patient. "I know many of these people aren't going to survive the year," Dr. Klein said, "but it's important to me and to them to preserve the quality of life they have for as long as they can keep going."

On another occasion, I visited the office of an obstetrician/gynecologist whom I had known in college. Frank Slattery was so glad to greet me that he invited me to take an im-

mediate tour of the clinic and its facilities. "But, Doctor,
what about Mrs. Jones, who's already prepared and in stir-
rups on the table, waiting for her examination?" his nurse
asked as we headed down the hall. "Oh, she can wait. I'll
be back in fifteen or twenty minutes," Dr. Slattery replied.
I was glad it wasn't my wife who was waiting.

I once sat in on the meeting of a medical-audit committee
of a community hospital. Its purpose was to review the
quality of care given in the hospital. The committee had
called on the carpet a member of the medical staff, an elderly
general practitioner. They were rightfully concerned that
two of his patients had died of heart attacks in the hospital,
without having been placed on the heart-monitor machines
that were readily available in the coronary-care unit. The
doctor was angry and defensive. He took refuge in the
"excellent care" he had given to thousands of other patients
over the last forty years. He refused to admit that he might
have slipped up this time.

One Thanksgiving Eve, a close relative of mine seemed
close to death in a nursing home. There was just a bare
chance she might respond to immediate, emergency medical
attention. I called Dr. Jim Smith, an internist friend of
mine, caught him just before he was leaving for a symphony
concert, and arranged for him to meet us at the hospital as
soon as the ambulance could get the patient there. Dr.
Smith, handicapped by a lack of adequate medical records
at that unusual hour, listened carefully to what I could tell
him, set up a program of transfusions and medications and
worked steadily with the patient through the night until
she turned the corner and began to live again.

To me, these experiences are worth remembering. They
illustrate that physicians are human beings like the rest of
us, even though sometimes they and we forget it. Most
doctors grew up with their fair share of prejudices, rigidi-
ties, and compulsiveness. I have met a few who are crooks
. . . and more who are saints. I have watched doctors make
three tough diagnoses in a row . . . and miss an easy one.

I have seen a tense, high-strung internist send patients away in tears when he was angry because one of his patients died . . . and heard him comfort other patients by phone from his home.

Doctors do protect their reputations, and their colleagues, as well as their patients. Many know their limitations; others don't. Most doctors keep up their education better than the rest of educated men and women. They read almost guiltily, go to medical meetings, and get consultations. Physicians in general are quicker than most to accept new ideas and to admit mistakes. The trouble is, medical mistakes are more costly than most.

That is all the more reason for you to have a clearer understanding of how the medical-care system works, its limitations, and how you can use it most effectively when you need it. The limitations of the system start with the failure of many patients to fully inform themselves about their health and to fully inform their physicians when they need medical care.

Walter C. Alvarez, M.D., former Mayo Clinic physician and noted medical columnist, summed up the problem from the doctor's point of view in this way:

> I still marvel at the way many patients who sadly need help, with great determination, withhold from their physician all of the information that he must have (1) if he is to make the correct diagnosis, (2) if he is to avoid making the wrong one and perhaps a disastrously wrong one, and (3) if he is to avoid wasting large sums on fruitless laboratory testing and perhaps a fruitless and unnecessary operation.

The physician's role isn't to judge what you have done or not done in terms of right and wrong, even though some physicians think it is. His job is, to the best of his ability, to get the kind of information from you that will help him make an accurate diagnosis and recommend therapy. If this is what you want him to do, be completely honest with him.

It's far better to say "I don't know," or "I don't understand the question," or "I'm not sure," than to give him a "yes" or "no" simply because you feel he is looking for a particular answer.

Even if you give the doctor full information, you have no guarantee that your illness will be correctly diagnosed and effectively treated. Keep in mind that more is still unknown than is known about what causes disease, how to prevent it, and how to treat it. The public tends to assume that physicians know most of the answers in the scientific age, because we have learned quite a bit about medicine from newspapers, magazines, books, and television. But modern medicine got off to a slow start only a century ago, and is just now coming of age.

Take the simple matter of colds, sore throats, and other respiratory infections. These are the most common illnesses for which people go to the doctor. Yet, by and large, no one knows specifically how to treat most of these infections. Fortunately, upper respiratory infections for the most part are self-limiting; that is, regardless of how you treat them, they'll be better in several days.

Physicians report that half of all the visits patients make to their offices are for conditions categorized as "not serious." Only 2 percent of visits end in hospital admission. But those 2 percent are the most costly, because the hospital has been the focus for most new advances that have been made in medicine and that are saving lives. Heart transplants and kidney transplants are only two of the more dramatic developments. Most hospitals now also operate coronary-care units and intensive-care units that save lives, but at higher and higher cost.

New drugs, too, have helped keep people alive longer. Our increasing longevity has created tremendous, costly demand for nursing homes and home-care services, services which have grown faster in scope and in cost than our ability to understand and control them.

It wasn't very many years ago that in most parts of the

country you could go to the doctor's office for four or five dollars. Now it's more like fifteen or twenty dollars for a visit; it's more, of course, for a house call (if you can get anyone to make one!) or a hospital visit. Hospital and medical costs have, in the last decade, risen much faster than the Consumer Price Index. If it weren't for the rapid growth of private and public health insurance, medical bills would rapidly dissipate the savings of any family in which a serious illness occurred.

Not long ago, a twenty-five-year-old secretary in an Eastern city developed a psychiatric illness. Her psychiatrist recommended that she spend some ten weeks in a nearby private hospital, with visits from him almost daily and the appropriate medications to speed her recovery (which eventually took place). The cost: $125 per day for the hospital, including drugs, and $25 per visit for the psychiatrist—a total of $150 per day, $1,050 per week, $10,500 for a ten-week period. Where does a twenty-five-year-old secretary find money like that? Obviously, she doesn't. Her health insurance, like most, covered only a small portion (40 percent) of her psychiatric hospital bills, and her parents, who lived across the country, had to take on the obligation. The mother went back to work and the family's plans for a new car, a vacation, etc., all went out the window.

It's no wonder—with the costs of medical care rising as rapidly as they are—that we get upset if something we are paying for doesn't go right, and it is easy to understand why most of us expect so much from our doctors. We think their knowledge should extend equally well into all areas of illness, and how to deal with it quickly and at minimal cost and inconvenience. Over the years physicians have unwittingly encouraged our belief that they are omnipotent and omniscient. Why is it that any of us respect a business associate or a lawyer for saying, "I don't know, but I'll find out," but we expect our physician to know all the answers? Doctors and patients both need to get over this feeling. Let's concede that doctors don't know everything, that they can find out some things that they don't know, and that they can admit, when it is true, that there isn't sufficient scientific documentation to be sure.

Next time you see your doctor, perhaps you'll have a healthier respect for both his knowledge and his lack of it. And next time, go with the awareness that your life and health are your own responsibility, not that of the doctor. Use the doctor and the rest of the medical-care system to help you make the most of your life and health. Finally, exercise these two vital rights:

1. You have *the right to know*. When your doctor makes a diagnosis or recommends a drug, a diet, or surgery, you have the right to know why and what it might mean for your future—both benefits and risks.

2. You have *the right to say no*. There is no law that says you have to do everything the doctor tells you. *Make your own decisions,* based on as much information as you can get. If you are uncertain, hold off taking a drug or having surgery until the doctor has fully answered your questions and you are convinced in your own mind that the recommended action will be the best for you.

With this new attitude, you can be ready to enter into a shared communication with your doctor, looking to him to *help you deal* with your health problems as effectively as possible.

2

CHOOSING A DOCTOR

CHOOSING A PHYSICIAN IS AN ART—NOT A SCIENCE. THE BIG-
gest mistakes most patients make in choosing a doctor are
these:

1. Choosing a physician on the basis of his personality
   alone.
2. Choosing a specialist to fit the ailment you *think* you
   have (self-referral), rather than choosing a primary
   physician who takes care of you as a person.

Personality in itself can be a deceiving factor. Of course, a
good many competent physicians have outstanding per-
sonalities; but every so often a physician will develop a following among patients—almost a worshipful following—
simply because of his personal magnetism.

I recall visiting the office of such a practitioner a few years
ago, and hearing him rattle off the names of his famous
patients as he took me through his suite of rooms containing
X-ray equipment, diathermy machines, and fancy labs. Two
factors destroyed my confidence in him very quickly: First,
many of his patients came back day after day, week after
week, for "special treatments" such as vitamin shots and heat
treatments, without even seeing the physician himself; second, his colleagues in the community were nearly unanimous

in criticism of his professional skills. While professional jealousy sometimes leads one doctor to run down another, it's usually a danger sign when a large number of physicians react similarly. Most doctors today have all the patients they want and a high degree of financial success, so that economic jealousy is seldom a factor in criticism of a colleague's professional ability.

Self-referral is another cause of unhappiness in choosing a doctor. You owe it to yourself and to your family to have one primary physician to call each time you are sick. Let him handle the diagnosis and treatment or refer you to the appropriate specialist when necessary. Otherwise you may be making continuing errors that can be costly in dollars, in health, and perhaps in terms of your life.

Not long ago a friend asked me how she should go about finding a new doctor for her family. Their family doctor had been stricken by a heart attack and they didn't much care for the young man who had covered his calls in recent weeks, so they had been sending themselves to the appropriate specialist when symptoms arose. That came to an abrupt halt when my friend developed a persistent backache. She first thought it might be due to a recurrence of an old kidney infection. So she called a urologist, who said, in effect, "That type of pain doesn't sound like a kidney infection. I'll try to think about it the way your family doctor might, but it's really not my line. Why don't you call an orthopedist?" After three visits and three X rays, the orthopedist was unable to pin down a cause. The woman, now confronted with a further choice among a gynecologist, a gastroenterologist, and a psychiatrist, decided instead to ask how to find a new family doctor.

As this anecdote illustrates, each person really needs a physician who is concerned about him as a whole person, not simply as a urologic problem or an orthopedic problem or a psychiatric problem. To benefit from the full range of services available in medicine, it's essential to start with a physician who is aware of all systems and organs in the body, how they interrelate, and how a person's day-to-day living patterns may affect them.

Almost any physician, on the basis of medical school and a couple of years of residency training, should be capable of providing this type of overall service. Many physicians, however, now go into such highly specialized training that their ability to deal with patients as human beings becomes clouded by their extreme interest in a particular organ or body system. And their experience limits them further.

At the other end of the spectrum is the physician in the emergency room of the hospital. He provides an element of primary care by being the physician of first contact, but he doesn't deal with a patient periodically over time. The primary physician cures both the lack of continuity and the lack of comprehensiveness in care. He or she is the person who concentrates on the continuity of the patient's life, in health and in illness, whether the patient is afflicted with a simple disease or with a complicated disease. In the words of John H. Millis, former president of Case Western Reserve University, "The primary physician is not defined as the physician of first contact, but as the physician who assumes the primary responsibility for the patient."

For the most part, the physicians best equipped to play the role of primary physician are family physicians, general practitioners, internists, and pediatricians. (These specialties are defined in Chapter 3.) Frequently an obstetrician/gynecologist can play this role for a woman during her childbearing years. Some physicians who are in subspecialties of internal medicine, such as gastroenterology or cardiology, still retain a strong interest in the patient as a person and like to perform the role of primary physician. Your choice will depend upon your personal preferences, the community in which you live, and the availability of physicians.

Here are some pointers that may be useful in determining which to choose:

1. If you are in your twenties or thirties with small children and want one physician to look after all members of

the family, the obvious choice is a family physician or general practitioner. He or she is trained to take care of problems from birth to death. He is able to cope with most problems of diagnosis and treatment, and he will refer to specialists those occasional problems with which he needs help.

2. An internist may be the best physician for you if your children are grown and you are middle-aged or older. These middle years often bring their share of chronic medical problems such as hypertension, diabetes, heart disease, and ulcer. As a rule, an internist is particularly well-qualified as a medical detective and a manager of multiple chronic illnesses. If he is your primary physician, he is more likely to refer you to another physician for treatment of certain diseases outside the specific area of internal medicine.

3. As noted, the obstetrician frequently acts as primary physician in providing care for women, although it is important to let him or her know that you are expecting that type of care. The pediatrician provides first-line care for children from birth through adolescence. Some pediatricians will also handle routine care for adults in the family, but this is not generally satisfactory for either the physician or the patient. The combination of pediatrician and internist works for some families.

In choosing a primary physician, don't worry about the label so much as his apparent ability to take care of your particular needs. If you are in an urban area you may find it more difficult as a rule to find a family physician as a primary physician. On the other hand, if you are in a rural area you will find it almost as difficult to find an internist. If you live in the suburbs you probably have your choice.

Consider also the type of practice of the physician. He or she may be practicing on his own; he may be in a partnership or group of two or more doctors of the same specialty; or he may be in a large multispecialty group. In any of these types of practices the physician should have an arrangement with other doctors to cover for him when he's absent and a willingness to consult freely with them.

1. *The solo doctor* offers the advantage of a continuing, highly personal relationship. You will see him consistently except when he is on vacation or away. He can come to know you so well that frequently a simple diagnosis and treatment can be handled by phone.

2. *A group of two to five family doctors or internists* offers the benefit that almost any time of day or night you can count on finding one of them available. The doctor you see regularly may well call an associate for consultation, sometimes at no charge to you. The disadvantage may be that you don't like to switch doctors, or that you don't care for one or more of your primary physician's associates. In some of these groups it's possible to establish one man as your personal physician and see him most, if not all, of the time. In others, the rule is that you must accept all physicians in the group and see whichever one is available at the time of your visit.

3. *The large multispecialty group* puts at your disposal a wide range of medical services—including a variety of specialists and a number of laboratory, X-ray, and other diagnostic services. Usually you can select an internist in the group as your primary physician and make your appointments only with him. He in turn will refer you to any specialist within the group (or outside it) if necessary. Often a clinic provides its own sophisticated diagnostic services, thus saving the patient from going elsewhere or into the hospital for expensive diagnostic tests. On the other hand, some large groups make it difficult for patients to see the same doctor regularly. You may feel that you're being treated on an impersonal, assembly-line basis. You may also feel that there is too frequent referral to specialists for consultations at an extra fee. These referrals may be a safeguard, but they have been overdone in some medical groups. Just don't count on a group practice being better per se than a single physician. A bad group—and there are such—is no better than a bad solo practitioner!

Once you've decided whether you want a solo family

physician or a group internist, how do you go about finding him in your community? The methods vary with the community and the types of medical services available there. By combining several of the guidelines that follow, you will improve your chances of finding the best physician for your family:

1. Call the county medical society and ask for the names of two or three family physicians, G.P.'s, or family internists in your neighborhood.

2. Call one or two of the telephone-answering services listed for medical exchanges and put the same question to them.

3. Call the hospital in your area, ask for the administrator's office, and put the same question to him or his secretary. When calling, make an effort to describe the sort of family medical service you require (number of children, ages, type of physician you have had in the past, any special problems, etc.). If the administrator's office is on the ball, you will be given names of physicians who might fit your particular needs—rather than just names from the rotating list. The latter is about all you will get from items one and two above.

4. Check with one or two persons in your community whom you respect. These should be persons who generally have good judgment and have lived in the community for some years, such as a banker, a lawyer, a clergyman, a business executive, a school superintendent or a principal. Seeking the advice of such a person, rather than simply asking a neighbor, can improve the odds of discovering the better practitioners in the community. If you have a few names to start with, based on the previous suggestions, you will be ahead of the game.

5. Check with related professional people, such as dentists, pharmacists, and nurses. One of the most reliable sources may be a nurse who has been working in the local hospital for several years. She will have had an opportunity to observe at first hand the level of patient care and the person-

ality of many physicians in the community.

6. If you're moving to a new community, ask your doctor before you leave your present hometown for the name or names of doctors in the new community. He may not know any personally, but he often can look up names of some well-trained physicians in your new home area.

7. If you do consult with friends and neighbors, one useful check is to find out the names of doctors who have cared for patients successfully through a long, serious illness.

8. Check with physicians themselves if you have the opportunity. If you know a general surgeon, an ophthalmologist, or a dermatologist, for instance, you might ask him which physician he uses for his family. It is sometimes (but not always) a satisfactory guide. Occasionally physicians themselves fail to have a primary physician!

9. When you call the hospital, get the names of those physicians who have been chief of the department of medicine or chief of the department of family practice in the last three to five years. These are men who are well regarded by their colleagues for their professional ability. Two hazards exist in this method: The physician who is at the top of his field locally may be so busy that he cannot take on new patients; and some hospital medical staffs may use a popularity system for electing chiefs, rather than a yardstick of competence.

Whatever you do, use three or more of the above approaches in combination. If the names of two or three physicians come up over and over again as you go through the checks suggested, you can be reasonably sure of their adequacy.

Should you interview the physician before you select him to look after you and your family? This doesn't hurt, but it's not likely to be profitable, since most physicians are not used to being approached this way, nor do most patients know what questions to ask. It is far better to go in with some routine problem, whether it be a sore throat or a camp physical for Johnnie, and get a chance to chat with the physician while you have a specific purpose in mind. You can tell pretty quickly whether his personality appeals to you. You should feel comfortable with him even though you've never met him before. A key question to ask yourself after your visit is: Would I feel free to ask this physician a foolish question? If the answer is no, then perhaps you had better continue your search. If the answer is yes, then you have found someone with whom you can develop rapport. Time will tell whether he will in fact provide the kind of medical care you and your family want.

3

WHICH SPECIALIST FOR YOU?

THERE ARE TWO WAYS TO ANSWER THIS QUESTION. THE FIRST is to divide specialists into categories of those you might choose yourself, such as a family physician, an ophthalmologist, or a psychiatrist, and those whom you probably will choose on the recommendation of another physician, such as an orthopedic surgeon, a gastroenterologist, or a radiologist. Among physicians in the first category, you will have to get as much information as you can on your own; in the second category, you can rely much more on the opinion of the referring physician. The other method of dealing with the problem of selecting a specialist is to gain better understanding of what the designation means and how to evaluate the credentials that lie behind it.

Most physicians today are specialists. The steadily decreasing number of general practitioners is being rapidly replaced by a new type of specialist, the family physician, whose training program of three years following medical school is now basically equivalent to the training program of several other specialties.

Under law, any physician licensed to practice may call himself a specialist regardless of his training or experience. In some parts of the country you may see ads in the newspaper or in the yellow pages for a plastic surgeon or a bariatrician (a doctor who specializes in weight loss). Beware of claims of specialization made by public notice. This is not a very reliable way to choose a specialist. Right now the best determinants for a specialist's credentials are these:

1. *Education.* To obtain an M.D. or a D.O. (Doctor of Osteopathy) license, every physician has to attend an approved medical school, whether in the United States or abroad, and complete a state or national examination. Beyond that, every physician today has completed one or more years of graduate training in a hospital internship or residency program. It is this segment of education that counts most in determining the qualifications of a specialist. From the doctor himself or herself, or from the Directory of the American Medical Association or the Directory of Medical Specialists, found in major libraries, you can determine whether a physician has completed a given number of years of training in his specialty, and where that training took place.

Unfortunately, since residency training has changed so much over the years, it is impossible to give any easy guidelines for judging the quality of a residency. Training for most specialties varies from three to six years; the locus of the best training programs is probably in a medical-school hospital for subspecialties, but for other physicians it may be as good or better in a community hospital. About all I can say is that lack of specialty training in a recognized residency is good cause to be suspicious of the label "specialist."

Evidence of continuing education is becoming more frequent. More than twenty states require participation in accredited education to maintain a medical-practice license; at least the same number of state medical societies have similar requirements for membership. So do some specialty societies. The AMA offers a Professional Recognition Award to physicians who voluntarily keep up.

2. *Specialty Board Certification.* Most but not all of the qualified specialists in every field have taken and passed certifying examinations by national specialty boards, such

as the American Board of Internal Medicine, the American Board of Surgery, the American Board of Family Practice, and the American Board of Psychiatry. There are twenty-two such certifying boards in the United States. All offer examinations regularly to physicians who have completed residency training requirements. Recertification is now the coming thing. The American Board of Family Practice requires its "diplomates" to be recertified every six years; other boards will soon have similar requirements.

3. *Specialty-Society Membership.* Almost all specialists belong to one or more specialty societies, ranging from the giant American Academy of Family Physicians (over 40,000 members) to tiny groups such as neurosurgeons or specialists in physical medicine and rehabilitation. Criteria for membership in these specialty societies is quite varied, and therefore no guarantee of capability. Some specialty societies require evidence that a member participates in a minimum number of hours of continuing education each year (a pioneer requirement of the AAFP), and all offer some national or regional courses to help members keep up. Lack of membership in one or more specialty societies is again a reason for suspecting the accuracy of a self-styled specialist label.

4. *Hospital Privileges.* This is the single most valuable way to evaluate a specialist. It relies on the judgment of his peers in a community; they not only elect him to membership on the staff of the hospital, but determine the extent of his privileges to take care of patients in the hospital departments to which he applies. For example, a well-qualified cardiologist will have full privileges to take care of all patients with cardiac disease without required consultation. A family physician or general surgeon frequently will have to obtain a consultant for some of his patients' cardiac problems.

More and more hospitals today are requiring that a physician be board certified in his specialty in order to get the specific privileges he requests. At times, too, these privileges are based on observation by senior members of the medical staff and on the results of periodic audits of the physician's work. However, the review processes in all hospitals are not the same. In some cases, privileges may be arbitrarily denied because the hospital already has too many specialists in a particular field, or the applicant has not received board certification. On the other hand, old-timers with longtime privileges in obstetrics or surgery are not likely to have those privileges removed even when they are no longer competent to provide specialty care.

5. *Experience.* Medical practice, as the term implies, requires experience to gain skill. A good part of residency training is devoted to "practicing" a specialty in the care of hospital patients. If a specialist doesn't keep up in his field with a sufficient number of patients, he can lose those skills in a matter of months or years. A highly skilled cardiac surgeon, practicing in an area where he has many competitors, may operate on only one or two patients a month, which is probably not enough to maintain his specialized ability. On the other hand, a family physician with some special training in cardiology, limited as it may be, may develop an unusual expertise because he is spending 25 percent of his time managing heart patients. (This is more likely to happen in a rural area in which a cardiologist or internist has not settled.) Experience is a good guide in picking a surgical subspecialist. You can find out, for example, how frequently a plastic surgeon has performed reconstructive hand surgery in the past two or three years.

Putting these elements together in choosing a specialist is not an easy task. The degree to which you should collect the facts and weigh them depends on the seriousness of the problem, and whether you are making the initial determination or relying on the advice of your primary physician. You can always ask him questions regarding the physician to whom he is sending you. If you are choosing a specialist yourself, the best single place to collect all the information is from the specialist's office; usually his secretary can give you answers by phone about his credentials and hospital privileges. But you may have to be persistent to get them.

Precautions to observe in selecting a specialist:

A medical-school doctor is not always the doctor you want. His appointment to a faculty position may be based on his ability to teach or to do research or to take care of esoteric diseases. He may not have the requisite skills to provide good patient care, or you may find yourself being used more as a teaching patient, examined by a host of young doctors, rather than being cared for in your own right.

A friend's recommendation can be misleading. He or she may not be familiar enough with your own medical condition to suggest the appropriate specialist. You may waste time and money before finding this out.

A specialist written up in a newspaper article is not necessarily the best choice. Some reports of new diagnostic techniques or treatments are misleading, or inapplicable to your own situation.

Following is a descriptive list of the major medical and surgical specialties with some clues to finding the right level of care in each case:

Family practice. This new, rapidly growing specialty is the first place many people should look for a primary physician. The American Board of Family Practice has been in business only since 1969, first certifying those general practitioners already in practice who wanted to gain specialty status and were willing to take board examinations. More recently, most board-certified family physicians have come from the new family-practice residency programs which now exist in about three hundred fifty hospitals around the country. The family physician is specifically concerned with continuing and comprehensive medical care for all members of the family, including health maintenance, diagnosis, and continuing management of disease, whether physical, psychological, social, or behavioral. His three years of residency training give him a strong base in medicine, pediatrics, and usually obstetrics. In most family-practice programs, some surgical training is also included. In addition, a new family physician learns to handle common psychiatric, dermatologic, or gynecologic problems in a family setting. Currently, this is the only specialty in which most of the residency training occurs in a "model office practice" which simulates the kind of world he will encounter later on. Other specialties, including internal medicine and pediatrics, still get most of their training in a hospital setting. Because of this, the family physician is perhaps better equipped to deal with common medical problems on a continuing basis, and is readier to refer the more difficult problems to another specialist—or at least to get a consultation.

Internal medicine. The internist has traditionally been distinguished as a diagnostician, and also as the manager of patients with chronic illnesses such as arthritis, heart disease, and diabetes. His training and temperament usually suit him to conduct a thorough investigation of the patient's complaint and to provide careful long-term care, both in the office and in the hospital. As the term implies, internal medicine is concerned primarily with diseases that affect the cardiovascular, respiratory, and digestive systems, where it is often difficult to find the sources of trouble. There are basically two types of internists—those who serve as primary physicians to adults, and those who serve as consultants for specialized conditions—although many do both. The major subspecialties of internal medicine include:

Allergy. An allergist adds one or two years of subspecialty training to his basic residency program in internal medicine. He deals primarily with respiratory allergy such as hay fever and asthma, and with gastrointestinal and skin allergies.

Cardiovascular disease. One of the fastest-growing subspecialties of internal medicine, this usually involves one to three years of additional training. Some cardiologists have become highly skilled technicians, using the diagnostic techniques of cardiac catheterization and sophisticated stress testing. In fact, some cardiologists now subspecialize within their own field. Some are best at inserting pacemakers; others at diagnostic work-ups; and others at long-term management of complicated cardiac problems.

Gastroenterology. Internists who have subspecialized in this area deal with ulcers, gallbladder disease, and other diseases of the digestive system. Like cardiologists, some have become expert in specialized diagnostic techniques and also work closely with surgeons in their field.

Other internal-medicine subspecialties. These include pulmonary diseases, metabolic and endocrine diseases, and malignant disease (oncology). As more sophisticated equipment and technology become available, many subspecialists choose to work only with certain types of patients and technologies.

Pediatrics. Most pediatricians spend most of their time taking care of generally healthy youngsters, monitoring their growth and development. Unfortunately, much of their training in a hospital setting emphasizes relatively rare problems which can be dealt with best by subspecialists such as neonatologists (who deal with problems of the newborn), pediatric allergists, or pediatric cardiologists. If you're looking for a general pediatrician, look for someone who has trained in a community hospital rather than a university center and/or who has been in practice long enough to learn how to recognize and deal with the common problems in bringing up children.

Obstetrics and gynecology. This specialty has the most difficult time deciding whether its practitioners are primary physicians or consultants. Too often, a woman looks to her obstetrician/gynecologist as her primary physician when he or she is not adequately trained or is not sufficiently interested to manage her care when a problem arises outside the female reproductive system. In general, younger specialists in this field tend to have a heavy obstetrics practice, and as they grow older do less obstetrics and more gynecologic evaluation and surgery. Because of the widespread use of birth-control pills and of estrogen replacement therapy in menopause, many obstetricians/gynecologists are well versed in practical endocrinology.

Psychiatry. More and more psychiatrists are entering practice each year, as the result of a heightened interest in this field. There is a trend in psychiatry today away from the Freudian type of analysis as a method of treatment. More emphasis is being put on the use of drugs for the treatment of anxiety, depression, and mental illness. More people are being discharged from mental hospitals and the stays in these hospitals are growing shorter. This offers more opportunity for the psychiatrist in office practice to treat patients with a combination of drugs and psychotherapy while they live at home. Many psychiatrists still feel themselves outside the pale of general medical practice, even though they have had four years of medical school and one year of general medical internship. The difference between psychiatrists and other physicians seems to revolve around the proportion of disease that is related to psychic as well as organic causes. In psychiatry as in other fields, there is a trend toward subspecialization, particularly in child psychiatry, adolescent psychiatry, and geriatric psychiatry.

General surgery. The general surgeon is the general practitioner of surgery. He is trained to do a wide variety of operations by the time he has finished his residency, yet in practice he is usually restricted by competition from surgical specialties such as gynecology, orthopedic surgery, and neurosurgery. The general surgeon as a result is likely to have a heavy concentration of abdominal surgery and vascular surgery—for varicose veins, as an example. The competition from specialized surgery may result in the general surgeon adding a certain amount of general medicine to his practice.

Surgical specialties. These include colon and rectal surgery (proctology), neurologic surgery, plastic surgery, orthopedic surgery, thoracic (chest) surgery, and urology. There is obviously a great deal of overlap among the surgical specialties. For example, hand surgery is performed by a variety of specialists, depending on the geographic—not physical—area: general surgeons, neurosurgeons, orthopedic surgeons, or plastic surgeons.

Eye, ear, nose, and throat. Nowadays, this field, which used to be covered by one specialist, is generally divided into two. The ophthalmologist takes care of the eyes, including refractions for glasses and eye surgery. The otolaryngologist takes care of the ears, nose, and throat, including ear infections, tonsils, adenoids, etc. There's a trend in the latter field toward subspecialization, with some practitioners dealing only with the nose (rhinology), the ear (otology), or the throat (laryngology).

Dermatology. It is said of this specialty that its patients never die, but never stop coming, because skin disease seems to be such a chronic, hard-to-eradicate entity. The dermatologist does some office surgery, such as removal of warts and moles. As a rule, if more extensive skin repairs are required, a plastic surgeon will be called in.

Pathology. This is a physician whom you will seldom see, but on whose talents you may be relying heavily. You will find him or her in the laboratory to which samples of blood, urine, and other body fluids or tissue specimens are sent for analysis. Depending on the results of these analyses, your doctor may confirm or change a diagnosis and course of treatment. The pathologist is particularly important in examining tissue specimens to determine whether or not these may be malignant, and in performing autopsies to ascertain causes of death. The latter helps physicians in the hospital to improve their ability in diagnosis and treatment.

Radiology. The radiologist may not be seen as frequently as some of his colleagues, since he may have a technologist taking the X rays when you go in for pictures. Much of the radiologist's time is spent evaluating X rays of various parts of the body, although he usually directs gastrointestinal series himself. These examinations may then be used by your doctor in making his diagnosis. An increasing

number of radiologists are putting their knowledge of X rays
to work in radiotherapy of cancer.

Other specialties. These include anesthesiology, neurol-
ogy, physical medicine and rehabilitation, and preventive
medicine. Doctors in the latter category work primarily in
public health or industry in an effort to improve the health
of large groups of people. Neurologists are involved in diagnosis of strokes and brain tumors, among other things.
Those in physical medicine and rehabilitation are playing
an increasing role in restoring useful function to those who
may be injured by accident or crippled by disease. Most of
the specialists in this category work in hospitals, as do anes-
thesiologists, radiologists, and pathologists.

4

THOSE NON-M.D. DOCTORS

Physicians guard their turf jealously, more so than most professionals. Among the invaders of the M.D. turf are other doctors practicing the healing arts: osteopaths, podiatrists, psychologists, dentists, and chiropractors. Sometimes they rival the M.D. in caring for patients; sometimes their specialized services are used by M.D.'s on a friendly, noncompetitive basis. Here's a quick rundown:

OSTEOPATHS

About 13,000 D.O.'s practice osteopathic medicine in the United States today, mostly in states that license osteopaths in the same manner as M.D.'s. Most D.O.'s are general practitioners or family doctors with less than 2,000 having other specialties.

On the average, the D.O. is about as well trained in medical school as is the M.D. who is a G.P. Colleges of osteopathy generally require a bachelor's degree or at least three years of college, as do medical schools, and provide a four-year course of training in most of the medical arts. Unfortunately, D.O. residencies for graduate training tend to be limited in quantity and quality, which has led some D.O. graduates to take specialty training in M.D. hospitals when possible.

Osteopathy differs from medicine in its emphasis on the relation of the musculoskeletal system to the total body concept. Osteopathic physicians add manipulative therapy to a combination of drugs and surgery to prevent disease or restore health. In manipulative therapy, the osteopath applies pressure to the bones, joints, muscles, tissues, and nerves as necessary to relax the body and stimulate blood flow.

In the past, the American Medical Association fought osteopathy almost as bitterly as it did chiropractic. But in recent years, the AMA has changed its attitude and recognizes that the quality of medical teaching in osteopathic schools parallels that in approved medical schools. In the state of California, D.O.'s were merged with M.D.'s in the early 1960's and efforts have been made to effect similar mergers in other states. A good many D.O.'s have resisted these merger efforts, as has the official organization, the American Osteopathic Association. Unfortunately for those who are seeking a physician experienced in manipulative therapy, the merger makes it difficult for patients to identify the D.O.'s. (Modern D.O.'s probably spend only 5 percent of their time giving manipulative therapy, much less than in the past.)

If you are looking for a D.O. in your area, check with the American Osteopathic Association, 212 East Ohio Street, Chicago, Illinois 60611, for the names of osteopathic physicians in your community who are members of the AOA. In at least fifteen states, osteopaths are on the staffs of M.D.-oriented hospitals.

PSYCHOLOGISTS

Many of these men and women offer diagnosis and treatment of mental and emotional disorders. Both the psychologist and the psychiatrist provide psychotherapeutic services. The training of the psychologist has a behavioral-science base and culminates in a doctoral degree, usually a Ph.D.

The psychologist is not permitted to engage in physical or drug therapy, as may the psychiatrist. He may, however, be particularly adept at the use of diagnostic psychological testing for children, adolescents, and adults. He should be a member of the American Psychological Association and be licensed or certified to practice clinical psychology.

Psychologists in private practice are concentrated in New York and California, with some growth in New Jersey, Illinois, Pennsylvania, Michigan, and Florida. Fees for psychologists generally run somewhat below those for psychiatrists in many areas. Their services may be covered by health insurance.

Your family physician may refer you or a member of your family to a clinical psychologist for diagnostic evaluation, and sometimes for psychotherapy. Psychiatrists are often unhappy about practice of psychotherapy by psychologists without collaboration of a physician. It's a good idea for anyone who is undergoing psychotherapy with a psychologist (or, for that matter, with a psychiatrist) to also be in touch with his family physician regularly, in case some organic problem needs attention. In choosing a psychologist, make sure you get a person with a doctoral degree whose training has included at least one year as a psychological intern in a mental hospital or clinic or who has achieved diplomate status with the American Psychological Association.

PODIATRISTS

Also known as chiropodists, these doctors carry the degree of doctor of surgical chiropody (D.S.C.), doctor of podiatry (D.P.), or doctor of podiatric medicine (D.P.M.). In a four-year podiatry college, following two years of undergraduate college work, the podiatrist learns manipulation, surgery, and prescription of corrective devices and special shoes to take care of foot problems. These range from ingrown toenails to tumors, growths, and abscesses.

Podiatrists are licensed in every state in the union, and in most states they now can prescribe some drugs and anesthetics. About one out of three podiatrists does some hospital surgery, always under the supervision of a physician. Many podiatrists are better at foot care than M.D.'s, particularly when it comes to those chronic diseases affecting the foot.

DENTISTS

Dentists are licensed in all states to do oral surgery, give anesthesia, take X rays, and prescribe drugs. About one in three dentists holds appointments at hospitals and, of course, works closely with physicians in those hospitals. Dental training includes four years of dental school and, more frequently now, one-year internships. A few dentists specialize in fields such as orthodontia, periodontia, oral surgery, and pediodontia. If you are looking for a dentist, many of the guidelines given in Chapter 2 will be of help.

OPTOMETRISTS

While a good many optometrists do not have doctoral degrees, more and more are receiving these as they complete five or six years of college-level study. Optometrists are also licensed, but only to prescribe and dispense glasses and contact lenses and to prescribe eye exercises. They do not have the right to prescribe medication, as do ophthalmologists. There is a distinct coolness between physicians and optometrists, for the most part. The M.D.'s feel that the optometrists have insufficient education to diagnose and manage visual problems other than simple visual defects. If you choose an optometrist to check your vision, it's a good idea to also have your family physician make a funduscopic and tonometric examination of your eyes when he checks you periodically. This way, if there is any evidence of disease that might be overlooked by an optometrist, your physician can catch it early. Some optometrists have developed outstanding reputations for eye exercises to correct childhood defects. When using an optometrist for this purpose, it is well to check out his reputation with your physician, or sometimes with the local school system.

CHIROPRACTORS

No evaluation of non-M.D. doctors would be complete without a mention of this controversial practitioner. Chiropractors are divided into two schools, those who stick to manipulation of the spinal column and those who have branched out into other methods such as electrotherapy, diet, and other modalities. Chiropractors are licensed in all but three states, but are not permitted to prescribe drugs in any.

While there are those who swear by the adjustments a chiropractor makes, there are others who feel that chiropractors are nothing but quacks. The American Medical Association feels strongly that chiropractic is a dangerous cult.

As a rule, the educational facilities for chiropractors are minimal, and in some states they are practically nonexistent. Gradually, state licensing laws are requiring certain basic science examinations or pre-professional college work prior to practice. This is removing a good many chiropractors from activity by their failure to qualify.

If you have heard of the values of manipulation, and you wish to seek this type of help, your best bet is to find a qualified osteopathic physician in your area and let him bring to bear his combined knowledge of manipulative therapy and medical diagnosis and treatment.

5

SHOULD YOU SEE A "PHYSICIAN EXTENDER"?

IN THE LITTLE TOWN OF DELTA JUNCTION, ALASKA, A HUN-
dred miles from Fairbanks, Ken Ryther, P.A., X-rayed and
examined the dangling foot of a little girl who had fallen
out of a tree, set the broken bone, and applied a cast in the
emergency room of his little clinic. Ken is a physicians'
assistant, one of a relatively new breed of "physician extenders" whose function it is to perform a variety of medical
and surgical tasks under the supervision of a physician—
in some cases, as with Ken, when the supervision is a hundred miles away in Fairbanks.

More and more physicians' offices now have physician
extenders, known as either physicians' assistants or nurse
practitioners. Nearly 6,000 physicians' assistants have gradu-
ated from 52 training programs accredited by the American
Medical Association. The total number of nurse practitioners is not known, because the programs vary so widely
and to date there has been little in the way of certification
or accreditation for nurse practitioners.

Physicians' assistants are neither unique to this country
nor new. The Chinese "barefoot doctor," the Russian
feldsher, and the African assistant medical officer are all performing similar functions in their own environments. Here

in the United States, medical corpsmen have served as physicians' assistants for years in the armed forces. But in the past decade, the demand for primary-care physirians, particularly for rural areas, has far outstripped the supply. Many young people—some returning from Vietnam with experience as medical corpsmen, and some with no experience—have been trained to become physicians' assistants in private office practices. At the same time, nurses have been getting additional training as nurse practitioners, equipping them also to perform more functions, particularly in pediatrics offices in rural areas. The advantages of these new physician extenders are:

1. They can be trained to handle commonplace illnesses under the supervision of a physician, who then can concentrate his or her own time on complex medical problems.
2. They can provide additional primary-care resources in areas of doctor shortage.

The training time for physicians' assistants usually ranges from one to two years, in addition to two years of college. The range of services provided includes taking histories and performing physical examinations; performing simple laboratory tests; diagnosing common problems; initiating minor medical or surgical treatments; assisting the physician in surgery; counseling patients, and their families, and writing prescriptions as ordered by the physician. Physicians' assistants in remote areas, like Ken Ryther, learn to handle a wide variety of emergency procedures to deal with auto accidents, heart attacks, and other emergencies.

When a physician extender encounters a problem beyond his or her competence, he or she consults with the supervising physician, in person or by telephone. Physician extenders who work alone in remote areas usually have a doctor visit their clinics on a weekly or monthly basis, to review the quality of the care, to see patients with complex problems, and to provide additional education.

Some studies of the use of physician extenders suggest that under proper direction, practice productivity increases 30 to 70 percent. In rural areas, this can be quite valuable. The physician extender also gives the solo doctor some relief from the twenty-four-hour, seven-day-a-week time pressures of practice. In most practices with physician extenders, patient acceptance has been quite high; the problem has been more with physician acceptance of these "in-between" practitioners. Some physicians feel threatened by a non-M.D. taking blood pressure or an electrocardiogram, taking a history, or writing a prescription. But with proper training and supervision, physician extenders have proven their ability to manage patient care successfully at a primary level.

Should you see a physician extender as your primary health provider? In a rural area, you may have no choice. There may be no physician available, or only one whose time is extremely limited. Chances are that the physician extenders in these areas rapidly become competent through "on-the-job" training, that is, through experience in diagnosing and treating a variety of common problems under supervision. The risk is that the physician extender may not recognize the signs and symptoms of an uncommon problem, or may not be sufficiently grounded in treatment techniques to handle a patient with several illnesses. So long as the physician extender recognizes his or her limitations and consults a physician in person or by phone, you have some safeguards. But the lack of recognition of such limitations can be dangerous. The only way to protect yourself in such a situation is to insist on seeing a physician—even if it involves some travel—if you are not responding to the treatment within a few days.

A further word of caution: Some nurse practitioners are seeking to establish themselves as independent health practitioners, without allegiance to or supervision by a licensed physician. This type of independent practice by a mid-level health practitioner is not likely to result in the best possible medical care. A nurse practitioner who does not function in an organized setting, affiliated with a medical practice or hospital, is more likely to make errors in diagnosis or treatment; furthermore, she or he is handicapped by not being able to use some of the diagnostic and therapeutic techniques available only to licensed physicians. Were the nurse practitioner working under the supervision of a physician, these techniques would be available by delegation.

6

HOW OFTEN DO YOU NEED A CHECKUP?

At age twenty-one, Molly Bright had to take a semester off from college to undergo back surgery. She then lived in a brace for several months. Molly had scoliosis, or curvature of the spine. This condition, if it had been detected when Molly was just entering her teens, probably could have been corrected without surgery and without loss of school time. Although Molly had regular checkups throughout her childhood, her pediatrician failed to detect the signs of scoliosis that must have been there when she was eleven or twelve.

Henry Bernstein, age forty-five, stumbled and fell during the second set of his weekly doubles game at a neighborhood indoor tennis club. He felt as if a giant steel band were tightening around his chest. Rushed to the hospital, he was placed in a coronary-care unit and fortunately recovered from a massive heart attack. The day before his tennis game, Henry had had his annual company physical, including an electrocardiogram, and was pronounced to be in good health. Reexamination of his pre-coronary electrocardiogram showed no significant abnormalities.

Both Molly and Henry were upset and angry. They had taken good care of themselves, had seen their doctors regularly for checkups, and then the roof had fallen in. They were ready to conclude that periodic checkups were a waste of time and money. Are they? I don't think so, at least not if you know what to expect from a periodic health examination and the doctor knows what he is doing. Don't expect life-saving miracles. Do expect that doctors will sometimes miss something. In Molly's case, her pediatrician should have detected the curve in her spine at one of the checkups she had at age ten or twelve. Had he used a simple technique of having her bend forward from the hips, he would have observed the hump that would have been present in her rib cage. This wasn't part of his routine then—though it is now!

During his checkup, Henry had had the kind of examination and advice that was right on target. It just came six months or a year too late. His doctor had told Henry that he had a higher-than-normal risk of heart disease because he was twenty-five pounds overweight, smoking two packs of cigarettes a day, and getting his only exercise once a week on the tennis court. Henry figured that if his electrocardiogram and blood pressure were normal, these cautions were not too serious. If something was wrong with his heart, it would show up on those tests. But heart-attack victims rarely have the kind of early warning signals that can be picked up on an electrocardiogram or in a physical examination. His doctor had done all he reasonably could have during the checkup.

The cases of Molly Bright and Henry Bernstein illustrate the rationale, though not the results, of periodic health exams:

1. Certain diseases can be detected early enough to prevent death, disability, or expensive, painful treatment.
2. Sound advice on better health habits, *if heeded,* can also prevent death, disability, or expensive, painful treatment.

Checkups will neither guarantee good health nor insure

against something serious turning up a week or a month later.

WHAT DOCTORS SAY ABOUT CHECKUPS

Physicians themselves have mixed feelings about the value of checkups. B. Leslie Huffman, M.D., former president of the American Academy of Family Physicians and a practitioner in Maumee, Ohio, considers giving sound advice on preventive maintenance to be one of the goals of periodic health exams. "If a man in his late forties in apparently good health comes in for a complete checkup," he says, "I sit down and review the five major risk areas for his age group: blood pressure, weight, elevated cholesterol, smoking, and diabetes. I tell him where he stands on each. When he is at risk, I explain why it is important to eliminate or control the risk factors and to return for monitoring."

Robert Manning, M.D., an internist and dean of the Eastern Virginia Medical School, Norfolk, sees other reasons for a checkup: "To assess the patient's health, to reassure the physician, to provide contact with the patient, or to reassure the patient that he is in good health." (The latter can backfire, as it did with Henry Bernstein.)

Francis N. Lohrenz, M.D., an internist at the Marshfield Clinic in Wisconsin, continues to do periodic examinations even though his own studies show that in one group of 375 management employees from a paper company, an annual physical "turned up serious undiagnosed disease—usually mild hypertension, mild diabetes, and the like—in less than 1 percent." Doctors are still faced with the necessity of performing "useless" physicals on many people in order to uncover a small number who have disease, he says.

"Medicine has taken the position that almost any amount of effort is justified if it results in the saving of even one life," responds Vincent R. Hunt, M.D., head of the Department of Family Practice at a hospital in St. Paul, Minnesota. "If we find a single treatable cancer in the rectum of an apparently healthy patient it makes the five hundred negative rectals done in the preceding three years worthwhile." But Dr. Hunt worries about being able to take care of enough sick people if he and his colleagues spend so much time searching for disease in apparently healthy patients.

There really is very little evidence on which to base the inclusion of all the specific tests that are performed in periodic health examinations. As Dr. Lohrenz says, "When a middle-aged patient we have regarded as healthy dies unexpectedly from a heart attack or turns up with terminal cancer, we guiltily wonder what we might have done to prevent the theoretically preventable. Our very human response is to keep ordering electrocardiograms, chest X rays, and sigmoidoscopies [bowel examinations] with only the remotest expectation that we will get positive findings." One study at the Mayo Clinic showed that it took about four thousand routine sigmoidoscopies to find *one* rectal cancer —at a cost of about $120,000 per discovery.

At the Milton S. Hershey Medical Center in Hershey, Pennsylvania, Dr. Joseph J. Trautlein, professor of medicine, wanted to find out which parts of the checkup—the history, the physical examination (done by the physician), laboratory tests, and X rays—were most valuable in checking a young and supposedly healthy group of medical-school freshmen. Of the abnormalities discovered among the 104 students who participated in the study, 40 were found as a result of the history, 16 from the urinalysis and a few other lab tests, only one from the physical exam, and none from the chest X ray. The conclusion: Most "healthy" young people don't need a costly health examination with a full battery of tests. But because of the high incidence of minor abnormalities, a screening exam consisting of a health history, urinalysis, and a blood test is definitely worthwhile.

While there is value in the early detection of some diseases, the major problem in the way of robust health for Americans is no longer disease itself, but rather the failure to adopt values of positive health. As individuals we face daily choices regarding diet, exercise, smoking, drinking, pill taking, to name a few, and as a society, we have made a number of collective decisions regarding control of life-style and environment. In Canada, the government has issued a report showing that the problems causing the greatest number of lost years of life are, in order: motor-vehicle accidents, heart disease, all other accidents, respiratory disease and lung cancer, and suicide. Most of these problems are not treatable by antibiotics or other *curative* therapies. But it is possible to control some of the factors in life-style and environment that increase the risks of dying from these causes.

That is why I think one of the more sensible (though not scientifically proven) approaches to periodic health examinations is based on the concept of health-hazard appraisal (HHA). HHA is a technique for assessing a person's individual risks of disease and death and relating the findings for the patient in such a way as to bring about a change in health habits.

More and more doctors are using this technique in their checkups. One such physician is Dr. David L. Hoff of the Family Practice Center in Akron, Ohio. He recently examined a forty-nine-year-old businessman, appraising his true "risk age" at fifty-four because of his health problems. The patient had a peptic ulcer and was fast becoming an alcoholic. His exam also revealed that he wasn't fastening his auto seat belt. Therefore, Dr. Hoff told him, his risks of dying from cirrhosis of the liver, from a motor-vehicle accident, or from pneumonia were higher than normal for his age. This gloomy forecast, however, could be improved if the patient would follow Dr. Hoff's health maintenance plan. He could reduce this "risk age" to forty-two, with a good chance of living longer than most others of his age, if he would stop drinking, use his seat belt regularly, and accept treatment for the depression that accompanied his alcoholism. A tough prescription, but a realistic use of a periodic examination to save a life or extend its usefulness.

If you are looking for a physician or a clinic using health-hazard appraisal, you can get a list of centers from Lewis C. Robbins, M.D., Director, Health Hazard Appraisal, Methodist Hospital of Indiana, Indianapolis, Indiana.

HOW OFTEN IS A CHECKUP ADVISABLE?

No one needs annual checkups from birth until death, even though this used to be the standard recommendation. It just hasn't proved to be valuable. The time interval between checkups should vary according to (1) the periods in your life: infancy and childhood, young adulthood, middle age and advanced age; (2) your family history; and (3) your own health status. For example, if one parent had diabetes, you probably should be tested for diabetes periodically.

Here is a schedule of periodic health examinations that generally applies. On pages 67–69 there are lists of details of the tests that should be included in the examination at various times.

Infants. Within twenty-four hours of birth, a thorough physical examination should be conducted. The pediatrician or family doctor should make sure that the baby has no physical defect that requires immediate attention, and that a correct classification of sex has been made. (Mistaken classification is infrequent, but any error that occurs should be corrected at once.) The physician should also order laboratory tests on the baby's urine and blood to check for errors of metabolism (the chemical changes in the baby's living cells). Just before the baby leaves the hospital, the physician should give him still another examination.

The baby's first visit to the doctor's office should usually take place between the ages of two and four weeks. By this time the baby's heart and lung systems have become adjusted to the work of breathing in the outside world. Defects in this system—which might not have been apparent in the first week of life—will now generally be noticeable. During this examination, the doctor not only will check the baby physically, but will also check his emotional and mental development and get a complete family history, that is, the details of the age and general health of the parents and any brothers and sisters. He will want to know about any allergies, physical defects, heart disease, diabetes, cancer, convulsions, mental illness, etc. This is the time to pick up any evidence of minimal brain damage that might impair the child's later development.

Each first-year checkup should include a brief physical examination of the baby, a history of any signs or symptoms of illness, a review of his habits and behavior, and a check of his measurements and temperature. Simple tests to determine hearing and visual ability should also be performed, and for girls a urine culture, which will reveal any hidden bladder infection, should be taken. Immunizations should be started during this time and should continue through childhood. The purpose of these examinations is not only to detect possible defects, but also to give the child the best possible chance to develop physically, mentally, and emotionally.

Toddlers. During the child's second year, checkups should take place every three to six months. At age three a thorough physical examination should be given, including tests for hearing, vision, and blood pressure, a blood test, and a tuberculin test. A complete dental examination should take place at the same age.

Children. From age three to age thirteen, a child should have a complete examination every two to three years, including tests for vision and hearing and appropriate immunizations. At age five he should be checked for possible color blindness. Do not rely on preschool and precamp physicals to fulfill this schedule, since they are often superficial.

Teenagers. During adolescence, a normal youngster need have a health examination only every four to five years (at about fifteen and nineteen). The physician will look for abnormal variations in physical growth, sexual development, and intellectual and emotional maturation. A boy or girl about to engage in competitive sports should be checked to see if he or she is physically ready for the stress of the game. The physician should look for any signs of a hernia, improper nutrition, skill difficulties, and glandular problems.

Young Adults. In the early twenties, the most significant medical problems, though they are not common, include menstrual disorders, fracture-risk factors, wound-risk factors, anemias, infections, head injuries, appendicitis, stomach ulcers, gallbladder disease, tonsillar disease, psychoneurotic disorders, and cancer. Most of these can be detected from clues in the history—that is, the series of questions about health asked by the doctor—or by a questionnaire such as that in Appendix A of this book, plus a limited group of lab tests.

Every young person about to get married owes it to his or her fiancé to have a health examination in advance of the wedding. Blood tests are not enough. A physical at this time may uncover defects or disease that both partners should know about. High blood pressure, for instance, is one of those silent diseases that particularly affect young men (blacks more than whites), and can cut five to fifteen years off their lives if not detected and treated early. Occasionally a young man or woman will find out for the first time about a heart defect that can be remedied through surgery, but which might otherwise lead to an untimely death.

While the period from twenty to thirty-four is usually the most healthy of adult life, it will still pay to have health examinations about every five to seven years, for these reasons:

1. *Early detection* of certain diseases that may strike younger people, such as cancer of the cervix, hypertension, or thyroid disease.
2. *Establishment of normal values* for future comparison. Since no two individuals have exactly the same set

of results from health tests, it's important to know specifically what the normal values are for you. Then if there is a change in these values the doctor can spot a potential problem quite early. Jack Reilly, who worked for a home-insulating company, had a chest X ray taken at age twenty-five that appeared normal. Another X ray taken at age thirty-five also looked normal. But when Reilly's doctor compared the two he noticed a minor change in one lung that clued him in to a possible work-related disease long before Jack had any symptoms.

3. *Early establishment of good health habits.* It's better to get on the right track in eating, sleeping, smoking, drinking, and exercise patterns when still in your twenties than when in your forties or fifties. Establishing good health practices early is the best way to prevent illness or minimize any disabling effects. Your doctor can help you with a program geared to your needs.

Of course, any person who develops symptoms such as a persistent cough, a lump or growth, hoarseness, signs of blood in the urine or stool, fatigue, headache, or specific aches or pains, should see a doctor right away without waiting for the next periodic health examination.

Middle-aged adults. Between ages thirty-five and fifty-nine, periodic health examinations should be conducted more frequently. If you are in generally good health and do not have a family history of diseases such as diabetes, hypertension, cancer, heart disease, or stroke, it may not be necessary for you to have a complete periodic health examination more than once every four or five years. Screening tests for hypertension and cancer should be done every two years or so. If you have a family history of one or more of these diseases, or if you yourself have been ill with something more serious than the run-of-the-mill cold or gastrointestinal upset, then it's probably a good idea to have a complete examination at least every two years from age thirty-five to age fifty, and probably once a year from age fifty on.

Statistics from a number of medical clinics and from corporations doing periodic health examinations on employees show that 90 percent or so of middle-aged or older persons having examinations do have some abnormality. Most of the time, the abnormalities are not really significant in terms of disabling or fatal illness. A laboratory test may show a borderline level of sugar or uric acid in the blood, neither of which requires intensive treatment, but rather observance of a carefully controlled diet and perhaps some weight loss. Other abnormalities may turn up in the history when the doctor asks about symptoms such as headache, tension, anxiety, problems in sleeping and in getting along on the job. Anxiety and depression are common disorders that can be treated.

Since the incidence of serious disease does increase with age, a periodic health examination in middle age often can unearth a major health problem early enough to do something about it. It may be an early cancer, early emphysema, some evidence of heart disease, or an early stage of serious mental illness. If the treatment is instituted early, a life may be saved or made more useful for a longer period of time.

An increasing number of corporations and labor unions are paying for examinations for employees or union members, in order to reduce the number of days lost from productive employment and to reduce the cost of illness and health insurance to an employer or a union.

Older persons. From age sixty to seventy-four, it's a good idea to have a periodic health examination once every two years, and from seventy-five on, once a year. This way you and the doctor can keep tabs on the general state of your health, including the progression of any degenerative diseases, such as arthritis, diabetes, or hypertension, and your mental and emotional health, as retirement ensues. Of course, he will also be seeing you if you do have any specific symptoms. Even if you do not—or if you think they are too insignificant to bother about—it's well to have at least regular reviews of the function of your body and mind. Nutritional counseling can be particularly important for the older person living alone.

WHERE TO HAVE A CHECKUP

In infancy and childhood the pediatrician or family physician taking care of your youngster should be doing the periodic health examinations. The problem is more difficult for adolescents. If your youngster has been going to a pediatrician, he or she may feel uncomfortable sitting in a waiting room with toddlers, and may wish to switch to your own doctor—whether you are seeing a family physician or an internist. A periodic health examination in the teens, say at entrance to senior high school or college, may provide the opportunity.

Otherwise go to your family doctor—be he family physician or internist. He is in the best position to provide follow-up when it is needed—particularly in helping you revamp health habits.

In case your family doctor is not interested in doing periodic health examinations (he may be so busy taking care of sick people that he feels he does not have time), ask him to suggest the name of another physician, usually an internist, who is known for his interest in periodic health examinations, or to suggest the name of a medical clinic in the area. Most clinics do have a regular program for such examinations, and many do them on a contract basis for employers or unions in the area.

In cities like New York, Chicago, and Los Angeles, special clinics have been set up to perform periodic health examinations for executives. Examinations performed in these clinics are usually of high caliber (and high priced). Their major clients are large corporations who periodically evaluate the results. If you are unsure about the thoroughness of your personal physician's exam, you can get a good crosscheck by seeing a medical clinic in your area for your checkup every other time. You will get some basis for comparison as well as providing your own doctor with another viewpoint about your health.

Whenever you consult a clinic or a physician other than your personal physician, make sure to request that a complete copy of the examination report be forwarded to him. Don't stop there. Call your own physician within a week or two after having the examination, and ask him if he has received the report and read it. Tell him you would like to come in for an office visit to discuss the results. (This will cost you an extra fee, but it's worth it.)

Finally, whether it's your own physician or a clinic that performs the examination, don't be afraid to ask the doctor who conducted it to interpret the results from start to finish. Don't expect him to give you every laboratory result numerically, since these may be confusing unless you understand the specific test and how it was performed. But you do have a right to know whether any findings were abnormal and, if so, what they mean in terms of your health. Since it is often difficult to retain this information, ask the doctor to give you a brief written summary, including any suggestions for follow-up.

COST OF A CHECKUP

In this field, as in most, you get what you pay for. Some "checkups" cost as little as $15–$25. Others cost $300–$500. As of this writing, you should expect to pay between $75 and $200 for an adult periodic health examination that includes a complete history, a thorough physical examination, a battery of laboratory tests, and additional diagnostic tests such as electrocardiogram, chest X ray, eye and ear exams. If the examination costs below $75, the chances are the physician cannot afford to spend the amount of time with you that he should in order to do a complete review. Nor is he likely to order all the tests that should be included, such as a stress electrocardiogram, or tonometry (for detection of glaucoma). If he charges over $200, the chances are he will include certain diagnostic procedures that may not be necessary for a routine checkup of a healthy person. These include X rays of the gastrointestinal tract, sophisticated testing of the heart and lungs, and specialized laboratory procedures.

Differences in cost relate in part to the variation in physicians' fees from one part of the country to another, in part to the amount of time spent by the physician and his assistants, and in part to the atmosphere in which the examination is conducted. Some executive health centers have plush surroundings, serve meals, and cater to executive tastes. The Greenbrier in West Virginia includes resort hotel accommodations for three days, for example. If this approach is to your liking, and you are willing—or your company is willing—to pay the extra cost, you can relax on the golf course between parts of the examination.

There is insufficient scientific evidence to justify complete physical examinations annually for any middle-aged adult who has no symptoms or signs of illness. Every so often, a lab test or X ray turns up a problem that otherwise would not have been detected until later; but whether early detection makes a difference is debatable, except in a few diseases. The major reason for having a *periodic* checkup is to focus on your own health habits.

COMPONENTS OF A PERIODIC
HEALTH EXAMINATION FOR ADULTS

TYPE OF TEST

HISTORY

Past medical
Family

Occupational
Psychological
Medicines
Symptoms review

PHYSICAL EXAMINATION

Height/weight
Blood pressure
Head
Eyes
Ears
Nose
Mouth/throat
Neck
Lungs
Heart
Breasts
Skin
Abdomen
Back
Neurologic
Extremities
Genital
Rectal

LABORATORY TESTS

Urinalysis
Complete blood count
  Differential smear
  Hematocrit
  Hemoglobin
  Stool (occult blood)
Blood chemistry
  Blood sugar
  Cholesterol

Tine test (tuberculosis)
VDRL (sexually transmitted disease)

DIAGNOSTIC PROCEDURES

Electrocardiogram, resting
Electrocardiogram, stress
Chest X ray
Eye examination
Tonometry
Hearing examination
Pulmonary function
Sigmoidoscopy
Mammography

MINIMUM PLAN FOR
PREVENTIVE CARE IN CHILDREN

Age	History and physical[1]	Height and weight	Developmental appraisal	Discussion and counseling	Physician's dental screening	Head circumference	Blood pressure
2-4 weeks	x	x	x	x	x	x	
2-3 months	x	x	x	x	x	x	
4-5 months	x	x	x	x	x		
6-7 months	x	x	x	x	x	x	
9-10 months	x	x	x	x	x		
12-15 months	x	x	x	x	x	x	
16-19 months	x	x	x	x	x		
23-25 months	x	x	x	x	x	x	
35-37 months	x	x	x	x	x		x
5-6 years	x	x	x	x	x		x
8-9 years	x	x	x	x	x		x
11-12 years	x	x	x	x	x		x
13-15 years	x	x	x	x	x		x
16-21 years	x	x	x	x	x		x

1 Observation of the undressed child, examination of the
mouth, upper respiratory tract, skin, musculature, motor
activity and behavior.
2 At this or next visit.

Vision	Hearing	Immunization	Tuberculin test	Hematocrit or Hgb	Urinalysis	Urine culture (girls)	Dentist's exam
X							
X		X					
		X					
X	X	X					
			X	X			
		X					
		X					
					X		
X^2	X^2		X	X^2		X	X
X	X	X		X		X	
X						X	
X			X	X			
X		X			X		

7

WHICH SIGNS AND SYMPTOMS REQUIRE A DOCTOR?

FAMILY DOCTORS REPORT THAT ABOUT HALF OF THE PROBLEMS they see in office practice are "not serious," according to the National Ambulatory Medical Care Survey. They rate only 17 percent of the problems they see as "very serious or serious," with another 35 percent being "slightly serious." In England, George Teeling-Smith, Director of the Office of Health Economics, says that "some people go to the doctor much too readily for quite trivial disorders, while others grin and bear it much too long." Here are a couple of examples that support his contention:

Arthur O'Malley, out for his Sunday golf game, stepped back without looking on the ninth hole; he stepped into a sandtrap, twisted his ankle and fell on it. His friends rushed him back to the clubhouse, put him in a car, and drove to the hospital emergency room. There the resident on duty felt the swelling, X-rayed the ankle, then told Arthur to go home and put ice on the joint and to wrap it in an elastic bandage before putting weight on it the next day. The cost: seventy-five dollars for advice that could have been obtained from any up-to-date first-aid book.

Howard Cardwell had just celebrated his fiftieth birthday when he had the first of a series of attacks of stomach pain, gas, and constipation. These recurred over several months, but Howard continued to get in to his hardware store, where he was under heavy pressure from a new chain-store competitor down the street. He figured the "indigestion" was just a result of business pressure. Finally, one noontime, when he couldn't touch his soup and sandwich, he stopped by his family doctor's office. A day later, after gastrointestinal X rays, Howard was in the hospital being prepared for surgery for removal of part of his intestine, which had become blocked by a growing cancer. Here was a clear-cut case of "grin and bear it" in the face of truly serious illness which he had chosen to ignore.

But wait a minute. Are these situations really clear-cut—or were they before you knew the outcome? In fact, the decision of when to see a doctor is much more complex than these case histories would indicate. Arthur O'Malley might well have cracked a bone in his ankle, requiring at least a light cast and the use of crutches. Howard Cardwell's stomach problems might have been simply the result of tension, and his investment in a visit to the doctor, plus X rays, might have been considered unnecessary. Both patients and doctors can sometimes judge symptoms to be more serious than they are—which results in unnecessary tests and medication—or they can miss truly serious symptoms, which results in failure to take curative steps soon enough. The latter is a more significant error than the former.

How can the average person tell when to call the doctor? First, there are emergency conditions which leave no doubt. In most emergencies, time is essential. *Don't waste it* by debating what to do next or whom to call.

Heart attack is the best example of an emergency in which time is truly vital. Dr. Lawrence Herman of Bellflower, California, reports that the average time between the onset of heart-attack symptoms and the arrival of the patient at a cardiac-care unit is four hours; but many patients do not live that long! Almost half of all coronary deaths occur during the first hour of the attack.

If you detect the signal of a heart attack, primarily a steady sensation of pressure in the center of the chest for two minutes or longer (some compare it to an elephant with his foot on your chest), get to the nearest hospital emergency room at once. Don't wait to call your doctor (unless yours is a small hospital with no doctor on the premises). If you are a friend or relative of someone who has such symptoms, don't discuss them: take action. Psychiatrist Thomas P. Hackett, M.D., of Boston, warns against the feeling "it can't be happening to me," or the reaction of a friend or relative who says "let's wait a few minutes and see how you feel." Says Dr. Hackett: "Teddy Roosevelt completed a speech despite having been shot in the chest because 'he knew it couldn't be serious.'"

Treatment for true emergencies is sometimes hampered by the "phony" emergencies that clog some hospital emergency departments. I don't mean the possible heart attacks that are not; I mean the sore throats, sore backs or stomachaches that people should have taken to the doctor's office or clinic during regular hours, if at all.

Fortunately, emergencies make up only a small portion of the illnesses or accidents that cause people to seek medical attention. The National Ambulatory Medical Care Survey shows that the two most common patient problems seen by family doctors in their offices are problems of the lower extremities (legs, ankles, and feet) and sore throat, followed closely by back problems, coughs, and colds. Others on the list: problems of the upper extremities (shoulders, arms, elbows, wrists, hands), abdominal pain, headache, fatigue, weight gain, wounds, problems of the face or neck, skin allergies, vertigo, and fever. If you have any of these problems, or others which are included in the list of symptoms on pages 75–81, here are some general guidelines to help you decide when to call the doctor:

1. *Report any recent change in health that is alarming or persistent.* Pain that comes and goes over several weeks, a lump in the breast or under the armpit, or blood in the

stool or urine are alarming enough to require seeing the doctor quickly. However, there are much less alarming changes that may also signal disease at an early stage. These include feeling tired all the time, having trouble sleeping, loss of appetite, unexplained weight loss, persistent hoarseness or cough, frequent headaches, stiffness in the joints on arising in the morning, etc.

It's easy to attribute some of these signs to getting older— but that is not necessarily the case. Some of these minor signs and symptoms, if they persist over a period of a week or two, may be indicators that your body is no longer functioning in the way it should. The range of problems indicated by each of these mild symptoms is so great that you run unnecessary risks should you decide to treat yourself for longer than a couple of weeks. For example, excessive fatigue may be a sign that you are not getting enough rest— or it may be an early indication of cancer, hypothyroidism, diabetes, or depression. Any condition which recurs over time should be checked out.

2. *Use common sense and drugstore remedies to treat a variety of common ailments.* The symptoms I am **talking** about now are the garden-variety cold, sore muscles from unaccustomed exertion such as gardening, swimming, tennis, etc., a hangover headache, temporary gastrointestinal upset, and other ailments which might best be described as self-limiting. At least 75 percent of illness is self-limiting and will clear up with little or no treatment. (The problem is to separate it from the other 25 percent!) As a rule, the only treatment a physician can prescribe is similar to that which you can prescribe for yourself: aspirin, bedrest, cough syrup, liniment, or another simple remedy. Don't be upset with him if he doesn't write a prescription for you. These forms of treatment are not cures, but relieve the symptoms until the underlying disease or injury has cleared up.

However, as the label on most over-the-counter medicine says, see your doctor if symptoms persist. As a rule, you can assume that if a cough, nasal congestion, or aching muscles or joints persists for more than ten days, the problem is serious enough for you to consult a physician.

3. *Consider the symptoms in relation to age.* In a child, persistent symptoms should lead you to consult a doctor sooner rather than later. Respiratory symptoms such as sneezing, wheezing, and coughing may be an indication of respiratory allergy. Repeated earaches may lead to loss of hearing. Headaches in a child may indicate some brain disturbance. Persistent irritability that is not characteristic of a child may point to any number of physical problems as well.

In a middle-aged adult, gastrointestinal symptoms may signal an ulcer, cancer, or gallbladder disease, among other things. Soreness and pain in back of the knee following a minor injury may indicate phlebitis (an inflammation of veins). Urinary frequency may signify diabetes, prostate disease, or a bladder infection. Frequent absences from work may mean a depression or perhaps alcoholism.

Caution: Once you know it is time to call the doctor, don't put it off! A national survey once determined that most people agree with most physicians on the conditions that should receive medical attention. These include:

Severe shortness of breath after light work
Unexplained loss of over ten pounds in weight
Cough of several weeks' duration
Lump or discoloration on skin, not a bruise
Unexplained constant fatigue
Frequent headaches
Diarrhea or constipation of about one week's duration
Rash or itch of one or more weeks' duration
Feeling of dizziness
Fairly frequent backaches

Having agreed that these conditions should have medical attention, the people who were surveyed then were asked if they themselves had had any of these symptoms. Many said yes, but admitted that at least a third of the time they had failed to seek out a physician.

The psychology of putting off a doctor's visit is understandable, but not always defensible in terms of your health. You say to yourself, "It'll go away," or "This is just something I have to get used to," or "This might be something serious and I don't want to find out quite yet."

Doctors themselves are just as poor in making decisions about their own health or the health of their families. One eminent cardiologist spoke before a major medical meeting in Chicago a few years ago, rushed to the airport in a cab, and as he waited to board his flight home, felt a strong pounding in his chest. He convinced himself that it couldn't be happening to him, managed to survive the flight to his home city, and took a cab to his hospital, where he spent the next three weeks in a coronary-care unit. Fortunately, he was one of the 25 percent who survived the four-hour period from the onset of symptoms until he reached hospital care. Next time, he says, he won't risk his life to avoid being thought a hypochondriac.

What about you? Your surest bet, if you think it could be an emergency, is to get help immediately. If you are not sure whether you need to see a doctor, call his office and report the signs and symptoms. If your doctor has well-trained personnel on the phone, they can help you make the decision. If you are sure that the aches and pains are minor and will go away—but they don't after ten days or two weeks—then see your doctor.

SYMPTOMS AND THEIR IMPORTANCE

SYMPTOMS	SOME POSSIBLE CAUSES	COMMENTS
Eating		
Belching	1. Overeating or eating too fast 2. Drinking too much 3. Alcoholic gastritis 4. Gallbladder disease 5. Ulcer disease	If associated with abdominal pain, see a doctor. If associated with a fecal odor, see a doctor promptly because

SYMPTOMS	SOME POSSIBLE CAUSES	COMMENTS
	6. Partial obstruction of the gastrointestinal tract 7. Wearing clothes too tight 8. Swallowing air	you may be developing bowel obstruction.
Drinking liquids to excess	1. Diabetes mellitus 2. Diabetes insipidus 3. Overeating of salty foods 4. Urinary tract infection 5. Compulsive water drinker 6. Drug overdose	If the person gets up at night to drink or has unexplained weight loss or urinary symptoms, see a doctor.
Loss of appetite	1. Depression or anxiety 2. Deterioration from arteriosclerosis 3. Chronic infection 4. Cancer 5. Hypothyroidism	Many children refuse to eat to control their parents. Watch for the teen-age girl who keeps dropping in weight and refuses to eat.
Nausea and vomiting	1. Gastroenteritis 2. Food poisoning 3. Pregnancy 4. Gallbladder disease 5. Appendicitis 6. Ulcer disease	If the symptoms persist more than a few hours, call a doctor. If the vomit contains blood, call the doctor at once—nausea and vomiting may also be the first sign of a myocardial infarction.
Overeating	1. Anxiety 2. Depression 3. Hyperthyroidism 4. Parentally induced habit	Once any hyperthyroidism has been ruled out, the cause is almost always emotional.

SYMPTOMS	SOME POSSIBLE CAUSES	COMMENTS
Eye Trouble		
	1. Refractive error and glasses need changing 2. Glaucoma 3. Allergy 4. Strabismus 5. Infection	Anyone experiencing persistent eye distress should be seen by an ophthalmologist. Watch for red eye that does not respond to treatment.
General		
Dizziness	1. Ear infection 2. Sinus trouble 3. Fatigue 4. Hypertension 5. Cardiac problems 6. Low blood pressure	Make sure the doctor takes the blood pressure and listens to the heart in addition to looking in the ear.
Fatigue	1. Depression 2. Hypothyroidism 3. Arthritis 4. Diabetes 5. Anemia 6. Cancer 7. Infection	This can be a very tough diagnosis.
Insomnia	1. Depression 2. Anxiety 3. Asthma 4. Congestive heart failure 5. Excess of coffee	In persons under 40 who have chronic insomnia, marital or family problems may be the cause.
Palpitations	1. Anxiety 2. Hyperthyroidism 3. Cardiac disease 4. Overuse of tobacco, alcohol, tea, coffee, "pep" pills	Always consider pills, and overuse of alcohol, tobacco, tea, and coffee before having a major work-up.
Trembling	1. Anxiety 2. Hyperthyroidism	Stop all drugs first. A neurologist may be

SYMPTOMS	SOME POSSIBLE CAUSES	COMMENTS
	3. Advancing age 4. Neurologic disease 5. Side effect from certain drugs 6. Parkinsonism	helpful here.
Weakness	1. See Fatigue 2. Myasthenia gravis 3. Anemia 4. Emphysema 5. Thyroid disease	
Hearing Trouble	1. Excess ear wax 2. Otosclerosis 3. Occupational hearing loss	Clean out the ears first.
Menstrual Problems	1. Anxiety/depression 2. Birth control pills 3. Cancer	
Mental/Emotional Anxiety	1. Psychoneurosis 2. Fear of serious illness 3. Drug reaction 4. Major life changes	Physical symptoms of anxiety include hyperventilation, dry mouth, palpitations, headache.
Depression	1. Personal loss (death, divorce, etc.) 2. Psychoneurosis 3. Organic disease 4. Drug/alcohol overdose	Depression often shows first in physical, not mental symptoms, such as fatigue, back pain, headache, dry mouth.
Memory loss	1. Senility 2. Hysteria 3. Drug/alcohol abuse	
Suicidal thoughts	1. Depression	Get help at once.

SYMPTOMS	SOME POSSIBLE CAUSES	COMMENTS
Pain		
Abdominal	1. Gastroenteritis 2. Stomach "flu" 3. Appendicitis 4. Ulcer 5. Gallbladder 6. Emotional 7. Cancer	If the pain persists or is associated with other symptoms, see a doctor.
Back	1. Usually muscular 2. Occasionally slipped disc 3. Anxiety/depression	Heat, rest, and a bed board take care of most back troubles. Don't rush to surgery.
Chest	1. Pneumonia 2. Coronary problem 3. Injury 4. Hiatal hernia	Severe or persistent chest pain should be considered a medical emergency. The same thing is true of abdominal pain radiating to the chest.
Face	1. Sinus trouble 2. Injury 3. Dental problem 4. Neurologic problem	"Tooth pain" sometimes turns out to be sinus trouble. Pain at the angle of the jaw may be related to the dental "bite."
Headache	1. Tension 2. Migraine 3. Sinus trouble 4. Brain tumor 5. Hypertension	An "uptight" person may suffer from migraine headaches.
Joints	1. Arthritis 2. Overactivity 3. Injury	If you are out of shape you may injure a joint quite easily. In addition to the usual causes, consider if this could be a serum-sickness-type reaction to a medicine taken one to two weeks ago.

SYMPTOMS	SOME POSSIBLE CAUSES	COMMENTS
Respiratory		
Coughing	1. Smoking 2. Pneumonia 3. Emphysema 4. Asthma 5. Cancer	A smoker who coughs should have a pulmonary-function test as part of his work-up, as well as X rays.
Shortness of breath	1. Smoking 2. Emphysema 3. Congestive heart failure 4. Asthma 5. Anxiety	If acute weight gain is also present, think of heart disease.
Sneezing	1. Hay fever (allergy) 2. Foreign body 3. Nasal polyps	Persistent sneezing and hay fever which do not respond to medication deserve an allergic work-up.
Wheezing	1. Asthma 2. Emphysema 3. Foreign body	All that wheezes isn't asthma, but most of it is.
Sexual Problems		
(including frigidity, impotence)	1. Decreased sexual interest 2. Failure to achieve orgasm 3. Fears and fantasies 4. Anxiety/depression	Counseling is important—with a doctor who feels comfortable treating such problems.
Skin		
Hair loss	1. Natural male baldness 2. Excess use of cosmetics 3. Emotional 4. Thyroid 5. Drug reaction	

SYMPTOMS	SOME POSSIBLE CAUSES	COMMENTS
Lumps	1. Benign tumors or cysts 2. Malignant tumors	Expanding, hard, bleeding, sore lumps are suspicious and should be biopsied.
Rash	1. Allergy 2. Infection 3. Manifestation of systemic disease 4. Drug reaction	If it persists, check with an allergist or dermatologist.

Urinary/Bowel Function

Constipation	1. Depression 2. Hypothyroidism 3. Diet 4. Bad bowel habits 5. Cancer	Constipation may be a symptom, a disease, or an attitude toward life.
Diarrhea	1. Food poisoning 2. Infection 3. Drug reaction 4. "Nervous stomach" 5. Ulcerative colitis 6. Cancer	Most diarrhea is benign and self-limited. If it persists and/or is associated with blood or mucus it should be worked up.
Urinary difficulties	1. Prostate disease 2. Bladder or urinary-tract infection 3. Diabetes 4. Anxiety 5. Gonorrhea 6. Anatomical problem 7. Kidney stone	A urinalysis and a rectal exam can diagnose many urinary troubles. Consider gonorrhea if any discharge is present in a sexually active person.

8

WHAT TO TELL THE DOCTOR

Dr. Clark Millikan, one of the nation's foremost authorities on stroke, has every elaborate piece of diagnostic equipment within his reach as a senior consultant at the Mayo Clinic. But Dr. Millikan, like all his medical colleagues, calls the history—not the equipment—the single most valuable tool in making a diagnosis.

The history is the data collected by the doctor about past and present—family illnesses, allergies, symptoms, and so on. Without this information, the doctor could spend thousands of dollars in testing before finding the cause of your illness. That's why, when you go to a doctor with a complaint, he starts the visit by asking questions. In a sense he is a Sherlock Holmes hunting for clues to the diagnosis. In this kind of detective work, little things can be very important, as the following brief case histories illustrate.

Harmon Brown, a sixty-two-year-old farmer, came into his doctor's office with his wife, assuring her and the doctor that he was just fine now. "What happened, Harmon?" the doctor asked. "I was coming in from the barn this morning when my arm became numb, then my leg and face. But I really feel okay now," said Harmon. The doctor moved into a series of questions: "How long did the numbness last? Have you ever had this happen before? Did the numbness start in one part of your hand and then move on up your arm? Could you use your arm when it became numb? Did you try to use it to pick up anything? Could you make a fist?" Harmon's answers to these questions gave his doctor sufficient data to decide whether the numbness was nothing serious, or whether it was a transient ischemic attack (a forerunner of stroke), was caused by a brain tumor, or had yet another cause.

Loretta Rose is twenty-nine, has three children, and is a very good housekeeper and mother. Her husband provides her with enough income to free her from household tasks part of the time, but she had to give up the career she had before she married. She recently visited her obstetrician for her annual checkup and Pap smear. On her way out the door she turned and said: "By the way, Doctor, I meant to ask you. I'm so tired when I get up in the morning. Can you give me some pep pills or vitamins?" The obstetrician had her sit down again and answered her question with more questions: "Are you just as tired in the evening as in the morning? How long have you been feeling so tired? Are you having trouble sleeping? Are you losing weight? Do you have any other symptoms? How is your husband doing now? How have the children been?" Loretta may have had a virus attack which left her feeling fatigued for as long as six to eight weeks. Or she may be suffering from what is known as "the tired housewife syndrome," a form of depression. Or she may have an organic disease such as alcoholism, anemia, diabetes, or thyroid disease. Her obstetrician was able to make a preliminary diagnosis from careful questioning.

In fact, Loretta was worried about Tony, her one-year-old. She had taken him to the pediatrician just the day before because he had had another of his "spells." "What are the spells like?" the pediatrician asked. "Does Tony appear to be holding his breath? Does he turn blue? Does he have jerky, uncontrolled movements? Does his body become rigid? What preceded the spell? Was he crying? Did he seem frustrated? Had you spanked him?" These questions helped Tony's pediatrician distinguish between an epileptic attack and a breath-holding spell associated with behavioral disturbance, something that, although frightening to parents, is not damaging to the infant and will usually disappear before school age.

Once the doctor has made a tentative diagnosis from the clues in the history, he usually seeks to confirm it through a physical examination, or with laboratory or other diagnostic tests. But he will almost always start with the history. In fact, there are many types of illness for which the diagnosis can only be made through the taking of a skillful history; even when other clues are needed, the history is almost always the key that unlocks the diagnostic door for the physician. Many a patient is not aware of this and either wittingly or unwittingly withholds information that could be of value to the doctor.

There was the case of Rosemary Weinberg, a shy, unmarried woman of forty who kept returning to her physician with complaints of digestive and abdominal troubles. A thorough physical examination and numerous X rays showed only slight abnormalities and could not account for Rosemary's widespread discomforts. Finally, the physician grew suspicious of her occasional weeping spells, and brought from her a reluctant "confession" that she had had three spells of unreasoning depression earlier in her life. When he asked why she had not mentioned these during her first visit, Rosemary said that she greatly feared that, if she told of her nervous storms, she would be committed to a mental hospital.

The doctor recognized something that the patient didn't know: depression may cause stomach upsets, in which case it is the depression that must be treated as the seat of the problem. Had she told him in the beginning about her depressive episodes, the extensive tests would not have been necessary. Her fears of hospitalization were unfounded; the doctor was able to treat her in the office with medication.

If, when you feel ill, you go to a physician who knows

you, chances are he will concentrate on a history of your present illness only. He will have in his files a record of your past medical history, of your family's medical history, of your psychological history, of your environmental history.

But if you are seeing a physician for the first time, or for a periodic health examination, he may want to cover all of these histories; others may have the histories taken by a nurse or medical assistant; still others may give you a printed questionnaire to complete by yourself. (A copy of one is included in this book.) Recently some physicians have used even more sophisticated techniques. One asks the patient to listen to questions on a tape recorder and to check off the answers on a special marking sheet. Another has the patient tap keys for "yes," "no," "don't understand" on a console as he or she watches questions flash on a television tube. No matter which technique is used, the physician himself should follow up by interviewing the patient in person. Don't expect that a mechanical device will replace the "detective's" pursuit of the possible cause of disease. It can only be an aid to get a uniform data base in a short period of time.

HISTORY OF PRESENT ILLNESSES

There are as many different questions, and as many ways of opening a medical interview, as there are doctors. Whatever your physician's opening question to you, come directly to the point and tell him (a) the symptom that is bothering you, be it pain, aching, burning itching, tiredness, anxiety, tension, the blues; and (b) what you think is wrong with you, for example, if you are worried that you have heart trouble, or an infection, or cancer like your mother.

It will be helpful if you have thought out ahead of time what you are going to tell the doctor. If you find yourself tongue-tied in the presence of the doctor, write your complaints out in advance. If you are describing a physical sensation, try to pinpoint exactly where you feel the discomfort. Whether the feeling is physical or emotional, describe when it occurs, how often, and for how long. Make sure to tell the doctor whether you have had similar symptoms in the past, and if so, what you did about them.

As the doctor listens to your description of the problem, he will be planning to follow up with questions about a certain area. He may ask if you are now taking any medications, since certain drugs have side effects that may imitate disease. He may ask if you have any allergies; and he may ask if anyone in your family has had similar problems. He will probably want to know if there are other symptoms that you haven't mentioned. For example, if you have complained of nausea and vomiting, he will want to know whether you have had diarrhea, loss of appetite, or heartburn. The combination of certain symptoms may add up to a diagnosis; even if they don't, they provide the doctor with signposts for his next steps in physical examination, laboratory tests, and other procedures.

Reminder: Tell the whole truth and nothing but the truth. You are using the doctor's technical skills and know-how to help solve your problem, not to leave your worries on his doorstep. If you want the most value from the time and money you are investing, don't hold back.

Like Rosemary Weinberg, some patients like to play guessing games with the doctor, concealing the true circumstances because of embarrassment, fear, a false sense of bravery, pride, or stoicism, or perhaps simply the feeling that it isn't important. If you are inclined to feel this way, keep these two points in mind: (1) Most doctors are not easily shocked or upset by any disclosures, no matter how private or bizarre they may seem to you. (If your doctor does react this way, you may want to get another doctor.) (2) Doctors are pledged to keep confidential any revelations you make, unless you authorize them otherwise. This is part of the doctor-patient relationship which goes back to the days of Hippocrates.

PAST MEDICAL HISTORY

If you are seeing a physician for the first time, he will want a detailed history of your past illnesses. This also can be written down in advance. His first concern will be for serious illnesses you have had in recent years, and particularly those likely to be chronic in nature, such as diabetes, arthritis, heart trouble, high blood pressure, migraine headaches, ulcers, or mental illness. He will also want to know whether you have had any allergies, drug sensitivities, or operations during your lifetime, and if so, which ones. Be sure to mention any hospitalizations for diagnostic reasons, even though no serious illness was discovered. Also tell the doctor about any physical handicaps, for instance if you are hard of hearing, or nearsighted, or have a limp, or have only one kidney. These facts form a background against which the doctor can superimpose information about your present complaints, or assess your present state of health if you are in for a checkup.

Mrs. Helen Morgan, a housewife in her forties, moved from Houston to a Chicago suburb not long ago. On recommendation of a neighbor she made an appointment with a local internist because she had been having intermittent abdominal pain. As part of the history the doctor discovered she had had her gallbladder removed three years ago. Mrs. Morgan also told him that she had had similar attacks of pain in the past after drinking a lot of fluids. These bits of information from the past enabled the doctor to rule out one cause of the abdominal pain—gallbladder disease—and to suspect another—kidney disease. He then centered his questions on other symptoms relating to kidney disease.

Tip: There is one question in the past medical history the doctor may not ask, but you should make a point of volunteering the answer if appropriate. Have you had recent dental work or dental X rays? Following dental work, infections may sometimes travel to other parts of the body through the bloodstream. This can be particularly serious if you have had a history of heart or circulatory disease.

FAMILY HISTORY

Knowing about major illnesses in your parents, brothers, or sisters can be as important to the physician as knowing about your own past medical history. Chronic diseases such as diabetes, heart disease, cancer, allergy, gout, and certain types of mental illness tend to be hereditary. If your doctor knows that a blood relative has had one or more of these diseases, he is in a better position to check you frequently for early signs or symptoms. Early detection of chronic disease may help the doctor improve your chances of living a reasonably normal and productive life.

A family history of communicable disease is also important. Tell the doctor if anyone in your immediate family —wife, husband, or children—has had or presently has tuberculosis or venereal disease. Both can be "silent" diseases (that is, without symptoms) in some people.

PSYCHOLOGICAL HISTORY

This is a tricky, difficult area. It is not easy to talk about your innermost thoughts and feelings; yet the doctor needs this kind of information just as certainly as he needs to know about your physical aches and pains. Sometimes illness is purely physical; sometimes it is purely mental or emotional; more frequently it's a combination of the two, with physical pain or illness being related to emotional or psychological factors. Ulcers, for example, are clearly physical in nature; they are painful sores in the lining of the stomach or duodenum. Yet ulcers seem to act up in response to emotional stimuli. Other emotional problems may result only in emotional symptoms. For instance, a person suffering from depression may simply feel blue and have trouble sleeping, may be unable to concentrate on the job, or even may have entertained thoughts of suicide. Yet depression is just as much an illness as an ulcer, and can be treated just as effectively.

Depression can be one of the most serious threats to your physical well-being. It can produce a variety of physical complaints that seem to keep changing; in fact, almost any physical symptom can mask depression. One of the most common is the feeling of a lump in the throat. Or it may simply be marked by fatigue, sleep disturbance, anxiety, loss of appetite, or just chronic unhappiness. In its more severe form, depression may lead to thoughts of suicide. At this point a person may feel that his life is hopeless, and that he would just as soon be dead. These are feelings which above all the doctor should know about, because depression can be cured.

Remember Loretta Rose, the tired young housewife? As her doctor began to separate functional or emotional causes from organic, he was looking for answers to questions such as these: "Do you have any particular mood problems? Are your spirits low at times? How serious do you think this is? Do you ever feel that life isn't worth living? Is there a particular stress situation that makes you feel worse?" In Loretta's case, the doctor did find signs of depression, and, over time, helped her to see how her feelings of boredom and frustration as a housewife and mother, and particularly her concern about Tony's spells, were causing her depression and in turn her fatigue.

ENVIRONMENTAL HISTORY

Finally, there is another kind of history that can be useful to the physician in helping his patients function more effectively, both at home and on the job. This is known as environmental history, covering details of your personal habits: smoking, drinking, exercise, sleep, diet, consumption of coffee and tea, driving habits, stresses on the job or in the home, leisure activities, and sexual life.

These factors can make a significant impact on your longevity and on your ability to enjoy life. Poor dietary habits or a too-stressful life-style may be the cause of physical symptoms. What's worse, they may lead to more problems ten years down the road. This type of history is the most important element of the health-hazard appraisal technique of health checkups, and forms the basis for a health maintenance "prescription" to improve your general health and sense of well-being. (See Chapter 6.)

A final word of caution: If you don't understand the doctor's question, *don't hesitate to ask for an explanation.* It's your health at stake, and that's important enough to make sure you know what's going on.

9

WHAT TO ASK YOUR DOCTOR— IN THE OFFICE

"WHAT DID THE DOCTOR SAY, GEORGE?"

"Something wrong with my kidneys."

His wife wanted the whole picture. "Exactly what?"

"I can't remember just how it went; he gave me some pills, and I'm supposed to do exercises."

"Oh," sighed the wife, "I suppose I'll have to call and find out for myself. If you don't know what's wrong, then you're not going to bother following his instructions—and I want to make sure you do."

How do you prevent this from happening? If you are the patient, make sure you understand everything the doctor said about your illness before leaving his office. Not only do you want to understand what the doctor said, but you want to make sure your own questions are fully and clearly answered. You have a right to know not only for yourself, but for those others who may be concerned about you.

Communication gaps between doctors and patients are commonplace, unfortunately—in part because the doctor and the patient are usually not operating on the same level. For the patient, this may be the first or second time to learn about a particular diagnosis or form of treatment; for the doctor, it may be the thirtieth time in the past month that he has gone through the same information. He tends to cover the ground rapidly because he is so familiar with it. It is like buying a house: most of us buy one only once or twice in our lifetimes, while the lawyers, real estate agents, and bankers we deal with go through the routines daily.

Dr. Lawrence W. Green, Head of the Division of Health Education at Johns Hopkins University, reports on several studies that show that "patients tend to be more dissatisfied about the information they receive from their physicians than about any other aspect of medical care. The evidence from a variety of sources clearly indicates that patients tend to under-report the amount of information they receive and the physicians tend to over-report the amount of information they give." Dr. Green believes that good communication between doctor and patient would be beneficial in a number of ways: speeding up the diagnosis, improving patient compliance with medication and other treatment, reducing unnecessary use of emergency services for symptoms that could be managed at home, reducing unnecessary appointments and telephone inquiries about misunderstandings, and even reducing unpaid bills and malpractice suits —which most doctors would love!

To illustrate Dr. Green's point about lack of communication, here is an excerpt from a roundtable discussion conducted by my journal, *Patient Care,* among several patients suffering from diabetes:

David Secular, college student: "The doctor doesn't seem to anticipate the questions and concerns that may be going through my mind as a new diabetic. When I ask specific questions, I get direct, thorough answers, but nothing is ever volunteered, and his answers don't anticipate what may be the next stage in an evolutionary process. The information comes in bits and pieces, sometimes after the time it would have been most useful.

"The specialist I go to gave me a book about diabetes that he had written. The trouble with it was that it had a chapter about the dangers of showing acetone, and I was showing a lot at the time. So, thanks to the book, I thought I was going to go into a coma, or blind, or something, right away. I have a lot of respect for my doctor, but I wish he would be more sensitive to the things about diabetes that are apt to bother people like me."

Marilyn Bonham, wife, mother, and psychotherapist: "When I first got diabetes at the age of nineteen, I was given a copy of Elliott Joslin's *Diabetic Manual*. The trouble was that my family doctor had ripped out all the pages that described the complications, which naturally made me very anxious."

Evelyn Brown, middle-aged housewife: "I first learned I had diabetes from my family doctor, but that is all I learned. He prescribed medication, but he didn't put me on a diet or anything, and I didn't ask any questions. I guess subconsciously I didn't *want* to know."

Mary McClellan, young housewife: "I want and need to know everything about my disease: what drugs I am taking and why, what my blood sugars are, what the other tests show. I want to know all the possibilities and what to expect, and if I do, I can handle anything."

Mrs. Bonham: "Diabetics want to know about insulin and syringes and bubbles and stuff like that, but when it comes to discussing the implications of being a diabetic for the rest of their lives, they run because they are afraid."

Mrs. McClellan: "But what can the doctor do about the reality of diabetes? Surely he can talk about amputation and blindness and hardening of arteries; but the only advice he can give is to take care of yourself on a day-to-day basis."

Mrs. Bonham: "I think he can do more. I think he can show you that he understands that you are suffering from a degenerative disease for which there is no cure, no possibility of any fundamental improvement, and with which there is the chance, even the likelihood, of one or more devastating complications occurring. It doesn't change the situation for the doctor to share this perspective with the patient, but it surely makes it easier for the patient to carry this knowledge if he has someone to say, 'I know how you feel.' "

This kind of understanding is the end result of good physician-patient communication, and requires cooperation from the patient as well as the doctor. Not every medical problem is as complex or as long-term as diabetes. But whatever it is, you will be able to cope with it better with an adequate level of understanding. Here are some practical guidelines to help you achieve a more satisfactory level of communication with your doctor:

1. *Write down your questions in advance.* Note down questions you may have about your symptoms—or about your illness, if it has already been diagnosed—or about your treatment. For example, if you wonder whether it's normal to be constipated after taking a certain drug that the doctor has prescribed, you will stand a better chance of getting an answer to this if you make a note ahead of time. Otherwise your repeat visit may go by with the doctor doing all the questioning and you providing only the answers.

2. *If you don't understand, say so.* The doctor has spent eight years getting his medical education and he has probably seen from a dozen to a hundred patients with a complaint similar to yours. He may lapse into medical jargon, or skip over explanatory points because he is so familiar with the problem. Many doctors think that every layman knows what a cyst is, or why avoiding salt may help you to lower your high blood pressure. If you don't understand words that he uses, or even whole explanations, remind him that you're not familiar with medical terminology or that he is going too fast.

3. *Ask for a full disclosure.* The physician may not always volunteer the facts, or may deliberately withhold them for the "benefit" of the patient. In some situations he may feel that the patient doesn't want to know. If you are the patient, it's *your* illness; you are entitled to complete information about the diagnosis, its implications, and the treatment.

Occasionally, the physician may suspect a psychosomatic illness, one in which a psychological problem may be causing physical symptoms, but may not want to say so. He may then prescribe a placebo—a pill that has no power as a drug—in order to test out his diagnosis. Obviously, if the patient knew he was getting a sugar pill, then the doctor's objective would be lost.

4. *Find out what shots will and won't do.* In this day of multiple immunization and vaccination treatment, every child and many adults expect an injection when they visit the doctor's office. Frequently the patient doesn't ask and the doctor doesn't explain what these shots are supposed to do, or what reactions might occur. Some shots are antibiotics or a form of vitamin. Others may be single immunizations against measles, mumps, or smallpox. Still others may be one in a series against typhoid, polio, or Asian flu. You will want to ask exactly what treatment or protection these shots offer or what they're supposed to do, how long their effects last, what side reactions may occur, and how serious these may be. Ask for, or make a written record of all shots for each member of the family.

5. *Ask for details on drugs.* Prescription drugs can cure a good many diseases or dramatically relieve their symptoms. They can also cause symptoms as annoying as the disease they are intended to remedy. Whenever the doctor prescribes a drug for you, ask him for its name, how it should be taken, how frequently, and for how long. Ask how the drug should help you, how it might affect you adversely, and how it might affect the action of other drugs you may be taking—or even your ability to consume alcohol, drive a car, or cross a street in traffic. Some drugs slow down your reflexes, make you drowsy. Others may have the opposite effect, leaving you jittery. Some drugs, particularly the barbiturates, can form a potentially critical combination with alcohol.

There has been increasing pressure for the government to require pharmaceutical companies to distribute "patient package inserts" describing side effects and adverse reactions for virtually all prescribed drugs, with the expectation that better patient education and protection will result. If such information were provided as standard procedure, and if the government requirements were not complex, it would simplify the job of the doctor in explaining the benefits and risks of a particular drug, and would reduce the number of questions a patient would have to ask—and the number of answers he or she would have to remember.

6. *Ask whether tests are normal.* Often a patient will have his blood pressure taken, or an electrocardiogram made, and from the bobbing needles on the machines will have no indication as to what is happening. Or he may receive a card with reports of laboratory tests on which he sees entries such as "cholesterol . . . 227" or "uric acid . . . 7.8." Don't make the mistake of letting a well-meaning friend or relative tell you what are normal readings for test reports. What is normal for him or her may not be for you. Norms vary according to age, sex, and ethnic background, and they vary according to how and where the test is performed. Only the doctor who knows both you and the laboratory can tell whether a reading is normal or not. So when a test of any kind is made, ask the doctor what the results were and whether, in his opinion, they fall within normal limits. Otherwise you may worry needlessly.

7. *Ask about restrictions on your activity.* Don't assume that the doctor knows that you play volleyball in the high-school gym every Wednesday, or do all your washing at home by hand. If he prescribes a course of treatment for your disease, ask him specifically about the physical activities you normally pursue (including sexual activity), and whether they will affect the treatment. Otherwise you may unnecessarily stop doing something for fear it might slow your recovery.

8. *Get it in writing.* Frequently the doctor may put you on a diet, outline an exercise program, or mention other forms of physical or mental therapy as part of your total

course of treatment. Ask him to put this in prescription form, just as he does for a drug he is giving you. Otherwise, after returning home, you may find that you've already forgotten points two and four. If the diet or exercise program is more complex, the doctor usually will have on hand a printed list or book describing specifically what he wants you to do. Don't hesitate to ask him for this kind of information. Or if you have already left the examining room, ask the nurse or receptionist before you leave the building.

9. *Do your homework.* Unless your disease is minor and of short duration, it would pay you to read up on it in a home medical guide or a library book. This type of background reading will enable you to ask intelligent questions. One caution: don't assume that *because* you've done your homework you know all the answers. Medical knowledge is advancing at such a rapid rate that medical opinion can vary widely; your own doctor may have a different point of view than you found in the book. He may also have some new facts at hand, or some information to challenge the latest "revelations" you may have come across in a popular magazine.

10. *Find out the forecast.* Sometimes a patient doesn't want to learn what the prognosis is. He or she may have the understandable but irrational feeling that if he doesn't know what the diagnosis means for the future, it can't hurt him, or it will go away. But many times a patient may suffer more from *suspecting* than from learning the truth. In the long run, asking about the future usually brings more peace of mind. Let the doctor know that you do want to know his opinion about the course of your disease. This gives him an opportunity to share with you not only his knowledge, but his hope.

In some practices, a doctor will introduce the concept of a "living will" (see page 98) as a means of opening up a discussion about serious illness. Dr. Lynn Carmichael, head of family practice at the University of Miami, Florida, tells patients:

"Both as a person and as a physician, my experience has been that a discussion in which a person calmly, openly, and freely expresses opinions and desires about the circumstances surrounding his or her death proves to be of inestimable value in times of stress.

"It enables doctors and nurses to know what the patient wants done in terms of life-preserving measures, and helps assure that the patient participates in critical decisions affecting his or her care."

Dr. Carmichael and his colleagues then provide a copy of a "living will," a document with no legal force, as a way of provoking discussion about dying and death, covering matters such as: What you wish to be known or not known; where you want to die—i.e., at home, in the hospital, etc.; whom you want to be present; and your feelings about such things as organ donation, burial versus cremation, and autopsy.

11. *Make it clear who else should know.* You have the right to privacy: without your consent the doctor will not inform your spouse, uncle, brother-in-law in Toronto, etc. If the doctor asks you whether or not you would like him to explain the situation to the relatives, consider when and whether you want this to happen. There are exceptions, of course, when children or minors are involved.

The days of the authoritarian doctor and the submissive patient are over. The patient has the right to know, and a right to participate in the decision-making about his or her health. Only by asking questions—and the right questions— can a person intelligently participate in this important decision-making process.

A *"Living Will"*
DIRECTIONS FOR MY CARE

I, _____, want to participate in my own medical care as long as I am able. But I recognize that an accident or illness may someday make me unable to do so. Should this come to be the case, this document is intended to direct those who make choices on my behalf. I have prepared it while still legally competent and of sound mind. If these instructions create a conflict with the desires of my relatives, or with hospital policies or with the principles of those providing my care, I ask that my instructions prevail, unless they are contrary to existing law or would expose medical personnel or the hospital to a substantial risk of legal liability.

I wish to live a full and long life, but not at all costs. If my death is near and cannot be avoided, and if I have lost the ability to interact with others and have no reasonable chance of regaining this ability, or if my suffering is intense and irreversible, I do not want to have my life prolonged. I would then ask not to be subjected to surgery or resuscitation. Nor would I then wish to have life support from mechanical ventilators, intensive-care services, or other life-prolonging procedures, including the administration of antibiotics and blood products. I would wish, rather, to have care that gives comfort and support, that facilitates my interaction with others to the extent that this is possible, and that brings peace.

In order to carry out these instructions and to interpret them, I authorize _____ to accept, plan, and refuse treatment on my behalf in cooperation with attending physicians and health personnel. This person knows how I value the experience of living, and how I would weigh incompetence, suffering, and dying. Should it be impossible to reach this person, I authorize _____ to make such choices for me. I have discussed my desires concerning terminal care with them, and I trust their judgment on my behalf.

In addition, I have discussed with them the following specific instructions regarding my care: _____

_____

_____

DATE _____ SIGNED _____

WITNESSED BY _____AND BY _____

10

WHAT TO ASK ABOUT PERSONAL PROBLEMS

"IN MY FAMILY PRACTICE," SAYS DR. THOMAS L. LEAMAN, A Pennsylvania physician, "many patients have questions about sex but do not ask them directly. They will ask the usual questions about contraception, about sexual relations during pregnancy, after surgery, or after a major illness, or about their children's sexual development.

"The more important questions, however, often go unasked. These questions are usually of a highly personal nature, involving the patient's concept of himself as a man or a woman, and are therefore emotionally charged. The problems often are hidden behind physical symptoms of illness, obscured by embarrassment, or completely buried, waiting for the physician to discover them."

These comments from a family physician strike home to people who, troubled by problems of sex, family relationships, mental illness, alcohol, drugs, or personal hygiene, may be too embarrassed to discuss them frankly with anyone, including their doctor. Medical, emotional, and social problems are often so intertwined that an individual may not be quite sure what's going on inside, and may be seeing the doctor for a physical problem such as insomnia, headache, or upset stomach, when the real problem is something else.

Not only is it difficult for the patient to confront personal problems directly in a session with the doctor. It is also frequently difficult for the physician to detect and treat these "hidden problems." Some physicians have a natural, often unconscious reluctance to become involved with patient problems that are complex, or that seem beyond their ability to solve, or that are sometimes just unpleasant.

How does one go about introducing one of these topics in the course of a routine visit to the doctor? It's not likely that such a problem would be mentioned when making an appointment; however, it should be possible to bring up the topic once one is alone with the physician—if he has your confidence—whether it's personal or concerns a close relative.

One technique is to make a brief written list of the topic or topics you would like to discuss, and go over this with the doctor. The Committee on Education in Family Life of the American College of Obstetricians and Gynecologists has prepared a patient checklist of problems, shown on page 106, which some obstetricians/gynecologists are now using. This list may be helpful to you in developing a way to present difficult personal problems to the doctor for discussion.

Ideally, a family doctor, internist, or gynecologist should be able to create a private and trusting atmosphere in which the patient feels at ease to express his or her concerns. But that will be true only if the doctor feels confident and comfortable in dealing with personal concerns and provides the means for communication. If a doctor appears to be making judgments, and expressing approval or disapproval, a patient will often feel turned off and unwilling to continue to seek help for these problems.

As a patient, therefore, you may have some feeling out to do on your own. If you feel uncomfortable discussing any personal problem directly with your doctor, it's best to explore some options, such as asking about which community, social, medical, or religious agencies might be best equipped to provide adequate counseling. Or ask your doctor to refer you.

Here are some specific suggestions for raising questions about the most common personal problems:

1. *Sex.* As Dr. Leaman noted, patients frequently ask about methods of contraception, or sexual relations during or immediately after pregnancy, or after illness, or about a child's sexual development. Any of these are good starting points in bringing up a more delicate question concerning sexual problems such as loss of potency, sexual frustration, or loss of libido (sex drive). Another approach is to use a general complaint such as, "My husband and I seem to be having problems with our sex life." If the doctor has an understanding of sexual problems and how to help resolve them, he will pursue this sort of statement with specific questions which are easier to answer than initiate. A third method of introducing the problem might be to ask if the physician can recommend an up-to-date manual on married love, or sexual adjustment. Again, the doctor is likely to pursue this request for information with additional questions to determine whether you have a specific problem in mind. If he does not, you are better off seeking advice from a counselor more attuned to sexual problems. The physician may be able to recommend such a person in the community.

The physician can be most useful if he has all specifics of the problem; he can't really help if you hide half the facts behind a curtain of embarrassment or false pride. Most physicians today are accustomed to handling quite specific questions about oral-genital contact, frequency of intercourse, painful intercourse, or inability to have an erection. They are not shocked or surprised by slang or by any common terms which may be used by a man or woman to describe an act or an organ; don't feel that scientific terms are necessary in describing your problem. Bernard Harpole, M.D., an Oregon family doctor, tells his patients: "I know all the words, proper or improper. You won't embarrass me or yourselves!"

2. *Marital conflicts.* Too often a husband and wife who are having trouble consider their problem unique, so that no one on the outside can have an answer except the divorce lawyer. This is not so. The family physician may be in a good position to discuss a marital problem, or certainly to refer a couple to a marriage counselor.

A not-infrequent approach is to say, simply, "Look, Doctor, I want to talk with you about my husband (or wife)." Another approach to discussing marital problems is through a symptom such as depression, anxiety, or insomnia. In his interview the physician is likely to give you an opening to express fears about your marriage.

3. *Other family problems.* More and more frequently the family doctor (or the local clergyman) is called upon to play the role of "surrogate grandparent," that is, the wise elder of the family who in the past was generally looked to as a dispenser of advice on all kinds of family and personal problems. With the increasing mobility of American families, most couples have no such elder statesman in the family to whom they can turn for personal consultations about child rearing, a "disgraced" relative, neighborhood problems, or even job counseling.

The doctor is often the best person to be seen when a family crisis arises. The pediatrician, for example, can resolve fears about the normal growth and development of your child. The general practitioner or internist can suggest alternative approaches to handling an elderly relative who no longer appears able to live alone. The obstetrician may be helpful in objectively pointing out the choices and risks faced by an unmarried pregnant teenager, her boyfriend, and their distraught parents.

When problems of this nature arise, even though they may appear to be nonmedical, don't hesitate to pose them directly to your physician. But don't expect the same kind of authoritative advice that you might receive on your strictly medical problems. In the latter case, the physician can usually prescribe a specific course of therapy for a specific disease. In the case of a family problem, he can help you best by being an objective listener and guiding you so that you find your own best solution to the problem.

When does such a problem in family relationships become serious enough to be taken to the family physician? When your usual solutions are no longer adequate: in other words, when you're upset enough so that no attempt at a solution seems to get anywhere. If you don't seek help at the point when you can no longer cope with the situation, your chances of having a physical or mental breakdown are dramatically increased. Perhaps the simplest example of this is the widow of a heart-attack victim who finds she can no longer cope with the burdens of bringing up her children. Grief over the loss of a loved one is natural and should require no extraordinary medical care. But when it continues to the point of becoming excessive, and interferes with the performance of day-to-day functions, then there is danger of falling into a depression which can and should be treated medically.

4. *Mental illness.* One of the most difficult problems to confront is the possibility of mental illness—anxiety, depression, paranoia, or one of the other types of neuroses or psychoses. Sarah Smith, age forty-five, with her last child going off to college, was waking in the middle of the night with attacks of unreasoning panic and fear. She dismissed these as bad dreams, but fortunately saw her family doctor soon after because she was having bouts of stomach pain and gas. In the course of the interview, she blurted out her concern over the panic attacks. After some further discussion, the doctor helped her see that these were part of a depression related to the "loss" of her children from the home and her feelings of insecurity as a person who was no longer an active mother. If you are concerned about feeling blue, crying a lot, getting uncontrollably angry, or any other mood problems, these can be expressed to your doctor

in just those terms. If he is sensitive enough, he will begin to ask further questions to determine how serious the problem is.

5. *Alcohol.* According to one series of ads run by a national committee on alcoholism, this disease affects almost everyone in the country either directly or indirectly. If you think someone in your family has a drinking problem, you may find that the doctor is your best adviser—that he may be a better person to discuss it with than disapproving members of the family or the drinker himself. The doctor should be able to review with you the way in which the family member drinks—when, how much, and why. From your answers, he can often tell whether you were right to suspect a drinking problem or not. One important clue is whether a person lies, alibis, and/or feels guilty about his drinking behavior. Another is that he drinks to relieve stomach pain or insomnia. A third is that he protects his supply of alcohol, even to the point of unnecessarily hiding it about the house.

Usually the physician will want the family member who drinks to come in. What can be done if you feel this person is going to refuse? The best answer is for the drinker's husband or wife to see the doctor for perhaps two or three visits. Doctors find that frequently a spouse unconsciously supports the behavior of the alcoholic partner. By counseling with the alcoholic's mate, the doctor may be able to bring about a change in his or her attitude toward the drinker. This in turn may result in the drinking partner becoming willing to make an appointment with the doctor.

An alternative is to encourage the drinker, himself, to make an appointment with the doctor for a physical examination. In any case, if you suspect a drinking problem, don't wait for the person to "hit bottom," as the old saying goes. Today, alcoholism can and should be diagnosed and treated at an early stage—before a person loses family, home, and job.

Caution: Not every physician is trained to diagnose and treat alcoholism successfully. If the physician takes a disapproving attitude toward drinking, it's better to seek help elsewhere—from another physician, a clergyman, or your local chapter of Alcoholics Anonymous. Chances are most physicians will use the latter organization as part of their program for helping to arrest alcoholism.

PATIENT CHECKLIST *

Listed below are topics about which many patients seek discussion. It will be helpful to your physician if you will check those you would like to talk about on this visit.

The checklist will be returned to you at the end of your visit.

_____Premarital counselling

_____Pregnancy

_____Contraception

_____Breast self-examination

_____Douching or other feminine hygiene practices

_____Menopause

_____Menstruation

_____Parenthood

_____Painful intercourse

_____Inability or difficulty in reaching orgasm

_____Homosexual feelings

_____Masturbation

_____Sterilization

_____Abortion

_____Doubts about whether or not you are normal

_____Difficulty in responding to partner

_____Finances

_____Sexually transmitted disease

_____Sexual inadequacy of partner

_____Marriage problems

_____Failure to please partner

_____Sexual practices

_____Divorce

_____Being single

_____Widowhood

_____Options in life-style

_____Pressures from friends

_____Social pressures

_____Loneliness

_____Security

_____Effects of medications, drugs, alcohol

_____Sexual assault, rape

_____Other (list)

* Prepared by the Committee on Education and Family Life and the Committee on Technical Bulletins of the American College of Obstetricians and Gynecologists, April 1977.

CHAPTER

11

"THEY SAY IT'S CANCER"

A FRIEND OF MINE FROM PENNSYLVANIA CALLED ME ONE DAY
with a plea for help. His sister Mary, who lived in the Southwest, had been told she had an inoperable cancer of the
colon. She had been receiving chemotherapy (drugs) to try
to knock out the spread of the cancer cells through her body,
with no apparent success. Her doctor then obtained an experimental drug through a cancer-research center, which
brought some apparent improvement—but it was only temporary.

"What hope is there for Mary?" my friend asked. Mary
was in her mid-fifties, married, with grown children. She
had accepted the diagnosis of cancer and the opinion that
she was not likely to live out the year. She didn't want to
use up all her husband's financial resources seeking cures.
But her husband didn't want to let any opportunity go by
that might result in a cure or remission—no matter what the
cost.

What advice can be given to a person, or family member,
when "they say it's cancer" or some other potentially fatal
disease? The first response is to say, "Any cancer is curable,
even though the odds may be against it." Statistics show that
even in lung cancer, which has the highest mortality rate,
chances are one in a hundred of survival after five years. The
chances of survival increase in relation to other forms of

cancer. So there is always hope, slim as it might be.

The second response I usually give is, "Has there been a second opinion?" Whenever a life is at stake, it seems unforgivable to me to settle for one physician's opinion, no matter how brilliant or famous he may be. In the case of cancer or another life-threatening illness, a second opinion should be sought from an expert in the particular illness, and more specifically, in the particular type of cancer (e.g., lung, thyroid, stomach). Your family doctor or the doctor making the initial diagnosis can arrange for such a consultation and should be willing to do so. If he is not, insist on it. Insist that he make the contact and provide all the pertinent data from the medical record to the consultant or to the consulting institution. The three best-known cancer research institutions in the country are M. D. Anderson Hospital and Tumor Institute, affiliated with the University of Texas, in Houston; Memorial Hospital, affiliated with Sloan-Kettering Institute for Cancer Research, New York City; and Roswell Park Memorial Institute, Buffalo, New York. Be aware, however, that sometimes a specialist will be quite willing to refer a patient to another oncologist (cancer specialist), but not to a specialty center. He may be afraid that the center will not return the patient to him after a consultation. Where a referral by a physician is required by the center, if the specialist refuses, simply ask your family doctor to make the referral.

There are also hundreds of competent oncologists at major teaching institutions around the country. These doctors often are better oriented to patients' needs than those at research institutes. Many of these physicians in a community setting are members of various chemotherapy study groups —for example, the Southwest Oncology group. If so, they have access to the same treatment protocols usually followed with the patients of the larger centers. About the only thing they do not have is access to the earliest stage of experimental drugs, which most patients are not interested in anyway. If the patient can establish that the physician is a member of one of these study groups, it would be another measure of assurance that the physician is considered competent by his peers.

If possible, ask your doctor to arrange a consultation with someone he knows and has confidence in, someone not too distant from your hometown, someone who can see the patient within a short time, and someone who is a specialist in the type of disease that has been diagnosed. Most family physicians, and certainly cancer specialists, are in a position to locate the right facility or individual. If you need further help, check with the American Cancer Society (or its local branch) or with the National Cancer Institute (a division of the National Institutes of Health), Bethesda, Maryland.

What form of treatment is best? Within the medical profession, there is still disagreement, and there probably will be until there is a high enough success rate in curing cancer so that most doctors will settle on one or two courses of therapy. Meanwhile, there are those who use surgery, or chemotherapy, or radiotherapy, or combinations of all three. Others also add psychotherapy. The decision depends on the type of cancer as well as on the doctor's inclinations and training. Almost every form of therapy seems to work with some patients, but not with most patients. Some have more distasteful side effects than others. Every year there are new experimental drugs and new methods of surgery and new methods of radiotherapy. So far none of these has been successful enough to become the dominant method of managing most cancers.

Should a cancer patient travel the United States or the world looking for a cure with experimental techniques? Some people have mortgaged everything they have to obtain treatments touted as cancer cures outside the United States. My friend from Pennsylvania said that he had heard of a new drug that was curing cancers of the colon in South Korea. Another friend with lung cancer was trying to track down a clinic in Germany that offered new forms of X-ray therapy in high doses. Chances are that each of these therapeutic approaches offers remission or cure to a few patients; sometimes spontaneous remission or cure occurs without therapy, too.

Only the patient and his or her family can determine whether to try the newest "cure." Unfortunately, the odds are *against* any one approach working. The costs of pursuing a variety of options are high—not only financially, but also mentally, emotionally, and physically. The only answer, I believe, is to decide how one wants to live out one's life. If the quality of life dictates going to any length to stay alive, the individual will pursue one or more long-shot options. If this kind of pursuit reduces the quality of life to an angry, frightened steeplechase ride, then the individual chooses not to go ahead.

I recall that several years ago a friend called me about her brother, who was dying of a rare form of lung cancer. Checking with my friends at several cancer-research institutions, I learned that there was an experimental new treatment for this type of cancer being used in England; with some effort, the treatment could be applied in the United States on an experimental basis as well. But my friend's brother decided against pursuing the experiment. He had already made his peace with himself, his family, and his God, and did not want to rekindle the candle of hope, on the one-in-a-thousand chance that it might continue to burn.

In such situations, the question often arises about continued hospitalization. More and more, persons with fatal illnesses want to die at home. The growing "hospice" movement in this country is developing home care as well as institutional programs for dying patients, usually with a hospital as a base. Specially trained nurses and other health professionals care for the patient on a regular basis in the home, and work with the patient and the family to help with the acceptance of death. Most cancer specialists know of hospice programs in their area.

Lack of insurance coverage for hospice programs has been a deterrent to their growth. But now Connecticut, one of the pioneer states in the hospice movement (which originated in England), requires health insurers to provide home health-care benefits to terminally ill persons who have six months or less to live, according to their physicians' prognosis. Such patients don't have to spend any time in the hospital to be eligible. Other states soon may follow Connecticut's example.

12

A POCKET HEALTH RECORD

No MATTER HOW GOOD A MEDICAL RECORD YOUR DOCTOR KEEPS, it stays in one place: in his office. This does you no good if you have an accident on the street, experience an emergency at home, pay a visit to a specialist, or fall ill in a strange city and have to go to the local hospital emergency room. Anne Simmons found this out when she moved a thousand miles across country to a new community recently. She sought out a new doctor after she developed acute bronchitis. After he checked her symptoms, he wrote a prescription for a drug called Polycillin®. Something about the name made her stop and think; she remembered that five years ago her previous doctor had warned her that she was sensitive to penicillin, which can cause severe reactions, even death. She asked her new physician if Polycillin® and penicillin were related. He came to attention quickly, said they were, and asked about her previous experience with penicillin reactions. Then he changed the prescription to an antibiotic not in the penicillin family.

Anne probably should have remembered to tell the doctor when she first saw him that she was sensitive to penicillin. The doctor certainly should have thought to ask Anne about her allergies or drug sensitivities. But doctors sometimes get so busy they forget to ask, and memory doesn't always serve patients either. In some cases, it can't. Peter Michaels, a seventy-year-old diabetic, was found unconscious on a park bench where he often sat to feed the squirrels. He was rushed to a hospital, where the emergency-room doctors figured he had had a stroke. By chance, his personal physician happened to be in the emergency room a few minutes later and reviewed Peter's medical history with the doctors on duty. Peter's problem was not a stroke, but a hypoglycemic coma, the result of the antidiabetic drug he was taking and a slowly developing impairment in his kidney function.

Fortunately, Anne Simmons and Peter Michaels survived, even though the facts vital to their health were between the covers of a medical-record jacket, filed and inaccessible to those who needed them at a critical moment of patient care. Others might not be so lucky. What can be done to make patient information more available when needed?

In our complex, mobile society, transfer of medical information becomes a difficult matter. Ideally, a nationwide computer program with terminals in every physician's office and in every hospital might give doctors immediate access to your medical history or mine. But this is not a very practical solution; the cost of developing and maintaining such a national data bank would be in the billions of dollars, if it were to cover more than 200,000,000 Americans on a truly up-to-date basis. Furthermore, any national computer-data bank would reduce the confidentiality of the information that is stored within it. I doubt that most of us would feel comfortable about having our medical records open to a wide variety of people, even if most of them are doctors. Unfortunately, any safeguard system for a computer bank seems to get broken within a few months.

Short of a computer bank, it is possible to have medical records move by mail or by hand from one doctor's office to another. If you are changing doctors, you should ask that your medical record be transferred to your new doctor, and the doctor you are leaving should be willing to do this. If you are seeing a specialist, you similarly have the right to ask him to send a copy of his findings to your family physician. In fact, it is a good idea to ask your family physician to send a summary of your record to any specialist you are seeing, so he has the full background on your medical history. If you are admitted to a hospital, your doctor usually supplies some medical-record information when he admits you, and the hospital usually sends a copy of its discharge summary to the doctor's office after you leave. But these exchanges don't always take place, nor is it easy for a patient to keep requesting various doctors to communicate with other doctors.

That's why I believe that the simplest way to transfer information is to have the individual be his or her own "computer medical-history bank." Since memory is unreliable, the best way to do this is through a personal health record which you can carry with you at all times and which contains the significant information that may save your life or avoid complications that can be painful and disabling.

Illustrated on the following pages is a "Personal Health Profile" that is adequate to give any health professional sufficient information to avoid many common errors in diagnosis or treatment. It is designed to be used by any family member, young or old, male or female. A set of "Personal Health Profile" pages are found in the back of the book. You can clip them out for use by each member of the family.*

To start your Personal Health Profile, fill in the Identification Data section. On your next visit to your family doctor, ask him to take a moment—while your medical record is on the desk in front of him—to complete the rest of the profile. He's in the best position to record the data correctly.

If you are seeing more than one doctor, ask the others, as you see them, to check the card for their own information, and to add any data that isn't included. Make sure you review it with any doctor you see, each time you see him.

---

* If you prefer, you can purchase the Personal Health Profile in wallet-sized card format, 5 for $2, from MILCOM, 322 Westport Avenue, Norwalk, CT 06856.

Then your Personal Health Profile will always be up to date. (It will be a useful guide, too, when you are getting telephone advice from a doctor.)

EXAMPLE OF A PERSONAL HEALTH PROFILE

On the following page is a filled-out Profile. Blank copies appear at the back of the book for your family's use. Here's how to make best use of the Profile.

Warning box: This is available for listing serious diseases, allergies or disabilities, such as epilepsy, diabetes, penicillin allergy, or use of a heart pacemaker. Your physician can best identify problems that should be stated here.

Identification data: Note the space for recording your health-insurance company and policy number. If you are covered under Medicare, that should be noted.

Problem list: Your doctor should list here all your significant problems. These include chronic diseases such as hypertension, diabetes, or glaucoma; major health events such as heart attacks or surgery; allergies; acute, recurrent infections; mental illness, etc. If the problem is still active, the "A" column should be checked. Otherwise the "R" column should be checked, meaning the problem has been resolved. A number should be assigned for each problem so that it can be related to the list of medications next to the Problem List.

Medications list: Equally important, this list can alert a doctor to suspect a drug reaction or interaction if you are suddenly ill. Your doctor should record the name of the drug, the dosage, and the date of starting and stopping. By problem number, he can indicate the reason for the prescription. The sensitivities section will alert him to problems you may have had with penicillin, sulfas, codeine, or any of the other drugs that often cause side effects. At the very least this section may save you an upset stomach; at the most it may save your life.

Spaces are also provided for blood type, so that should

you need a transfusion this can be handled appropriately, and for vision prescription, in case you wear glasses or contact lenses that need to be replaced quickly.

PERSONAL HEALTH PROFILE *
Carry this with you at all times.
Review with your physician at each visit.

WARNING!
I (am) (have) __Diabetes__

Identification Data:

Name __Susan Smyth__

Address __1010 First St.__

City __Anytown__ State __Mt.__ Zip __00000__

Home Tel. __101-222-1111__

Health Ins. Co and No. __Genl. Ins.Co. #2222-00__

In emergency, please notify:

Name __John Smyth__ Tel. __(office) 555-4444__

Physician __Dr. S. Wills__ Tel. __555-1111__

Prob. No.	Significant Problems	Status		Prob. No.	Medications	Dosage	Dates	
		A	R				Start	Stop
1	Diabetes	✓		1	Diabenese	250 mg.	8/14	
2	Hysterectomy		✓					
3	Urinal tract infection		✓					

A=Active   R=Resolved

Sensitivities
to medication **Sulfas**

Blood Type: **A+**   Vision Rx: **None**

13

HOW MUCH ATTENTION SHOULD YOU EXPECT FROM YOUR DOCTOR?

SOME YEARS AGO I USED TO SEE AN OPHTHALMOLOGIST WHO HAD an excellent clinical reputation for refractions and general eye care. But I walked out of his office in disgust one day and didn't return for five years. I had been waiting forty-five minutes past the scheduled appointment time, and had a business appointment which I was going to miss if I had to wait ten minutes more. I finally picked up my briefcase and left when his secretary responded to my latest inquiry with, "I know the doctor will just be a few minutes, Mr. Miller. But I can't tell you just how long. Please sit down and wait." It was the fourth time in two years that I had cooled my heels in this doctor's waiting room, and I had had it. I was not the only one. Many other patients had reacted similarly; they too resented being kept waiting with no adequate explanation nor any idea of how long the wait would be. As a result, his practice began to dwindle. Fortunately he recognized the problem, obtained some competent advice, and began to run his office on schedule.

The doctor's use of time in relation to his patients is important to him and to you. To him, time is an economic factor, since in his office, time is the commodity for which he receives his fees. He has to juggle emergency, urgent, and routine demands to handle an office full of patients and keep up with those in hospital beds and in nursing homes. And he still wants some time left for his family and his personal interests. To you, the doctor's time is something you want most at moments of great need, such as when someone in the family is seriously ill or when you have an acute problem. Then you want an instant response—by phone, or in the office, or even with a house call. Here are some considerations that can help you make the most of the time available to you and give you an understanding of what you can expect in medical-office efficiency:

1. *Getting an appointment*

Depending upon how sick you are and which doctor you're trying to see, it may take an hour or six weeks to get the face-to-face attention you're looking for. The wait is particularly long for appointments with certain specialists such as ophthalmologists, otolaryngologists, and psychiatrists. Some specialists in internal medicine and surgery now schedule weeks ahead for relatively routine examinations. These lengthy delays in most cases can be attributed to a shortage of such specialists in a given area.

On the other hand, a family physician, general internist, pediatrician, obstetrician, or dermatologist usually recognizes your medical needs when you call and schedules you accordingly. Their appointment books are less likely to be filled for months or weeks ahead. If they are, it's a sign that a practice is overloaded and the doctor probably shouldn't be accepting any new patients.

The best way to get an appointment in a hurry is to tell the doctor's receptionist when you call that there is an emergency. Describe it to her. No matter how far ahead he is booked, and unless he is unwilling to accept new patients, each physician has enough extra time in his daily schedule to fit a true emergency. Even if your problem is not an emergency but is urgent (for example, an extremely painful joint) you should be able to get an appointment the same or the next day.

It's important to let the receptionist know as much as possible about your problem so that she can convey this information to the doctor, and at the same time try to schedule you as quickly as possible. She holds the key to his appointment book, and can be a valuable ally. But if she tries to block you out, insist on talking to the doctor directly.

2. *Waiting time*

Some years ago, a survey published in *Medical Economics* Magazine indicated that three out of four patients with an appointment had to wait more than fifteen minutes to see their doctors. One out of four had to wait more than thirty minutes, with an appointment. Nine out of ten patients without an appointment had to wait more than fifteen minutes, and one out of two had to wait more than half an hour.

Why the delay?

In some cases it's legitimate—when caused by an emergency. Such an emergency can be of two types—the result of an accident, or the result of a discovery in the course of routine diagnosis that the patient has a bleeding ulcer or is threatened with a heart attack. Naturally these emergencies require extra time and effort on the part of the physician and his office staff; they cannot be anticipated, and most people are understanding about delays of this nature.

Other reasons for delay, some of them more understandable than others, include: tight scheduling of patients and a very busy practice; telephone calls with patients, hospitals, and other doctors; too much time-of-day conversation with patients; personal business; and the variable time needed to treat even a routine complaint. Diagnosing and treating an upper-respiratory infection, for example, can vary from three to twenty minutes, depending on the patient and his or her medical history.

What can you do about it?

First, you can accept a reasonable wait as something relatively common in most physicians' offices—and by reasonable we mean about fifteen to thirty minutes. Drs. Walter Lane and Wayne Lafferty, family physicians in Temple Terrace, Florida, found in a study of two thousand patients that they averaged forty-five minutes in the office from the time they entered until they left, including treatment time. If you plan on a forty-five-minute total visit, you won't schedule another appointment too quickly or you won't plan on picking up the children after school and seeing the doctor, all within a half-hour period.

Second, you can check with the receptionist when you arrive to determine about how long the wait will be. If it is likely to be more than thirty minutes, it's very much in order for you to ask why, and whether it's possible to reschedule the appointment at a time when the doctor can be reasonably sure of seeing you on schedule. The best way a doctor can know that you're unhappy about a delay is if you tell his receptionist. Some doctors who get tied up in surgery or with an emergency have their receptionist telephone patients to give them notice of the delay and a chance to change appointments. An excellent idea!

Third, you can ask the receptionist what time of day is least crowded on the doctor's schedule. If you can arrange your own schedule to fit these times, you may find that your wait will be substantially reduced.

3. *Treatment time*

Most doctors on an appointment system allot ten-, fifteen-, or thirty-minute segments to individual patients, according to their type of practice. Whatever the time segment, it does not truly represent the amount of time spent with each patient. Part of it may be devoted to routine checking performed by his office nurse such as blood pressure, electrocardiogram, collection of a urine sample or a blood specimen, or preliminary questioning that will give the doctor more information when you see him personally. Doctors Lane and

Lafferty learned that this preliminary data collection most often took three minutes, but could vary from no time to thirty minutes.

Though the doctor may not spend a full ten or fifteen minutes with a patient, he may be spending that much or more total time on the patient's problems. (Doctors Lane and Lafferty averaged eight minutes per patient in their practice study.) Remember that he has to review your medical record before you come into the treatment room. He may also have to interpret the results of laboratory tests or an electrocardiogram. He may need to talk with a physician consultant—or the family—about your problem. After your visit he must always spend at least a few minutes putting the pertinent data on your record for follow-up. He may also have to complete insurance forms or review your X rays with a radiologist.

Interruptions to watch for: the doctor who has four or five patients in different treatment rooms, and runs back and forth from one to another instead of dealing fully with one patient before going to the next (alternating between *two* patients is often an efficient use of time) . . . the doctor whose nurse feels free to open the door and interrupt while he is examining or talking with the patient . . . the doctor who accepts non-emergency telephone calls while in the middle of examining or treating a patient. For the most part these interruptions are unnecessary in a well-run medical practice. You should not hesitate to let the doctor and/or his receptionist know that you are disturbed by them.

4. *Advice by telephone*

How available is your doctor by phone? There's nothing more frustrating than waiting hours for the doctor to call back, when the receptionist or telephone-answering service has said, "I'll have Doctor call you," and then hangs up.

If it's an emergency situation, you should expect a call back within fifteen minutes—either from the physician himself or from another doctor who is covering for him. To get this kind of response, however, it is imperative that you let the receptionist or answering service know how critical the situation is.

If it is urgent but not an emergency, such as fever and vomiting in a child, you should expect a call-back within an hour—again, as long as you make the situation clear to the person at the other end of the phone. Don't insist on speaking to the doctor; it makes more sense to spell out the problem, ask the receptionist to repeat it, and find out just how long it will be before the doctor will call back.

In most other situations, and unless you have good reason to ask for a quick follow-up, you should expect the doctor to return your call within two to four hours.

What can you expect from your doctor when you get him on the phone? In an emergency, you can expect quite specific and complete advice on the immediate steps to take. Otherwise you should not expect the same kind of service by phone that you would receive in his office.

Most physicians can follow up a course of treatment by telephone, evaluating symptoms and their improvements on the basis of having seen you previously. Prescription renewal or change in drug, diet, or other therapy can be made by phone, in some cases without a repeat office visit. On the other hand, most doctors are correctly reluctant to make a diagnosis by phone, particularly if they have not seen the patient in some time. Obvious exceptions to this are upper-respiratory infections or gastrointestinal infections at a time when these may be prevalent in the community. But, for the most part, the physician needs to evaluate the physical signs of illness as well as the symptoms that may be described by the patient.

Should you expect the doctor to dispense routine advice on child rearing or family problems on the telephone? Some patients use their physician as "a member of the family" to discuss the kinds of everyday living problems that everyone has. Most family doctors and pediatricians are willing to fill this role—to a limited extent. Therefore, it's a good idea to be brief on the phone; if the problem is complex, make an office appointment. Most doctors are reluctant to charge for telephone advice, and most patients are not eager to pay for it. Perhaps if more doctors did charge for telephone time as they do for office time, patients would be more careful about asking for it.

Telephone habits that may bother you: the doctor whose phone is busy most of the time . . . the doctor whose receptionist never lets you get through to him . . . the doctor whose receptionist promises a quick call-back and then doesn't keep the promise. You have every reason to let your doctor know if you are bothered by poor telephone manners such as these.

5. *House calls*

Do doctors still make house calls? Yes, but infrequently. You're fortunate if you can find a primary physician in your area who will come to the house when it's necessary. If you live in a small city or town, your chances of finding a doctor who makes house calls are better than if you live in an urban or rural area. In the suburbs it depends—on the suburb and on the number of doctors available.

Nationally, family doctors and pediatricians average no more than two or three house calls a week—less than half the number they made twenty years ago. The reasons for the decline are these:

a. The shortage of doctors has increased the patient load that each practicing physician carries today. He can see four or five patients in the office in the same hour that he might spend on the road seeing two patients.

b. Though the physician traditionally charges more for a house call than for an office visit, his house-call charge doesn't really compensate him for the loss of productive time in his office.

c. Even more important, the physician on a house call

can't do as thorough a diagnostic work-up as he can in his office or in the hospital emergency room. His black bag can't deal with laboratory tests or electrocardiograms that are extremely valuable in diagnosis and treatment.

Assuming you can find a doctor who does make some house calls (and you can learn about this by asking his receptionist when you call for an appointment), when are you justified in asking for a house call? As a rule of thumb, the justification these days must almost always be medical. This means that the doctor should be the one to make the decision in view of the patient's condition, the need for diagnostic or therapeutic facilities, and the competition for the doctor's time. If you want the doctor to make a house call, your best bet is to explain the symptoms or signs of the illness as clearly as possible, such as fever, dizziness, pain, etc. Indicate any problem there may be in transportation, and then ask: "Is it possible for the doctor to make a house call, or should we try to get into the office?"

Which types of patients are most likely to get the house calls that are made? The elderly patient with chronic disease, who requires home-nursing care and is not strong enough to make the trip to the office. As a rule the doctor feels he can do more for a sick child, even when fever is present, if the parents bring him to the office. (The fever won't get worse from an auto trip, even on a cold day.) He prefers to send patients with acute chest pain, serious difficulty breathing, abdominal pain, or head pain directly to the hospital, where emergency treatment can be mobilized rapidly. Of course, your chance of having the doctor make a house call is also improved if he knows you and knows that you would not be asking for such a visit needlessly.

When the doctor makes a house call, don't expect him to turn it into a social visit or a checkup for members of the family other than the person who is seriously ill. You'll not see him at your home again if that happens! Give him the freedom and privacy to examine the patient as though he were in his own office—without a cluster of anxious relatives hanging over the bedside.

In the future you may see more house calls being made by allied health professionals working for a physician. Some doctors now use medical assistants to visit chronically ill patients at home to check their progress, to change dressings, to provide physical therapy, to check on medications, diet, exercise, etc. In some cases, pediatric assistants or nurse practitioners are making well-baby visits to the home of newborn infants. This gives the doctor information about the family life in relation to the baby, and makes care of the infant easier for the new mother. These allied health personnel in all cases report back to the doctor, who maintains final responsibility for care of the patient.

6. *If your doctor is unavailable*

It's becoming more and more rare to find doctors who are available to their patients twenty-four hours a day, seven days a week. There are still a few such physicians in practice, working their way to an early grave or at least a nervous breakdown. For the most part, however, the typical doctor works about fifty-five to sixty hours a week. This includes the time he sees patients in the office, in the hospital, in nursing homes, and on house calls. It also includes the time required to complete medical records, insurance forms, and hospital records; to keep up with his continuing medical education through reading, consultations with colleagues, and attendance at lectures and clinics.

As a rule, most family doctors make hospital rounds in early morning, see office patients during the day, and clean up any house calls or additional hospital rounds in late afternoon or early evening. Their work week sometimes includes Saturday morning office hours (for which a mid-week break is taken in compensation) and availability for night calls from three to five nights a week. Chances are that most primary physicians will be off call two or three nights a week and every other weekend. Other specialists may take more time off.

Because of the doctor's limited availability, it may be well for you to choose a partnership or group to provide your family medical services; coverage is then available twenty-four hours a day. This way you can get to know at least one other doctor and he or she can get to know you. In addition, this physician will have access to your medical records should your own doctor be unavailable.

If your doctor is in solo practice, find out from his office whether he has a regular arrangement with one or more of his colleagues in the community to cover for each other. Make a note of these doctors' names and phone numbers and try to see them at least once on a relatively routine visit. Then if your doctor is unavailable and an emergency occurs, you and the doctor covering for him will at least have had some personal contact preceding your call. Suppose you haven't been able to make these advance preparations and find your doctor is unavailable. If you can reach his office, ask the receptionist to give you the name of a physician who is covering for your doctor. You can put the same questions to the doctor's exchange operator if his office is closed. If neither alternative works, call the hospital and ask the operator the same question. If necessary, ask the hospital operator to connect you with the emergency room, which keeps a list of physicians and the men who have agreed to cover for them during their absence.

The emergency room is becoming more and more popular as a place for people to go when their own physician is unavailable, or for people who do not have their own physicians. Most hospital emergency rooms today are staffed around the clock, or at least have a physician on call who can be there in a few minutes. Small hospitals, those with under 100 beds, tend to rely on attending staff physicians—that is, private practitioners—to be available in the emergency room periodically. Larger hospitals just as frequently staff the emergency room with residents or interns, or with physicians on contract, whose primary purpose is to handle the emergency services in the hospital. Many of the patients using emergency rooms do not have urgent problems, but seem to prefer the hospital setting to a private practitioner's office, particularly when night or weekend hours are not available in the office. Use of the emergency room is advisable only when there is a true emergency, or when you feel that a problem is extremely urgent and your own physician cannot be reached. Otherwise, it is frequently a less than satisfactory method of obtaining routine medical care; the waiting times are lengthy, the costs are high, and the quality of care varies according to who is staffing the emergency room and the overall load of patients at any given time.

7. *Hospital visits*

The time that any doctor spends with his hospital patients varies widely according to their illness and his role in their care. These are guidelines to what you should expect if you or a member of your family is hospitalized:

If the problem is surgical: The surgeon should make a thorough examination, which may take from thirty to sixty minutes or longer, prior to his final decision to operate. You should also expect a brief visit from the anesthesiologist prior to surgery, and if your primary physician is continuing to supervise your care, he should be seeing you for from ten to thirty minutes prior to the operation. After surgery, the surgeon and/or family physician, depending upon who is responsible for your post-operative care, should be seeing you once or twice daily for from five to fifteen minutes to check on your progress and to answer your questions. If possible, request that your family physician or internist be the primary doctor responsible for your care.

If the problem is medical: The amount of time required of the physician in the initial stage of care will vary widely according to the severity of illness. In some cases an internist, pediatrician, or family physician may spend four or five hours in constant monitoring of an acutely ill person. But normally the initial visits are from fifteen to sixty minutes. Once the acute phase of illness is over, you should expect the same type of brief, daily visits mentioned above.

Remember that the physician spends additional time relating to care of the hospital patient beyond the time at the bedside. He will normally spend five or ten minutes a day checking and completing hospital records and writing orders for the nurses regarding a specific patient. He also expects to spend time talking to anxious relatives from day to day, particularly during the acute phase of illness and just prior to the time the patient is discharged.

If the doctor is not checking his hospital patient at least once daily, chances are that the patient no longer needs the full services of a general hospital; he might be served as well in an extended-care unit, a nursing home, or at home, with less frequent visits and less supervision by the physician.

14

HOW CAN YOU TELL
IF YOUR DOCTOR IS GIVING
YOU GOOD CARE?

ROSA ORTIZ, A WORKING MOTHER IN HER THIRTIES, RUINED her resort vacation on the second day by taking a tumble from a rented motor bike. She burned her leg on the hot metal of the bike muffler, and after a restless night, went to the local hospital emergency room for treatment. The doctor on duty cleaned the burn, applied an ointment, and gave her a prescription and written instructions on care of the wound. On her return home five days later, the burn was still painful and oozing; Rosa went to her family doctor, who prescribed a slightly different course of therapy with no better results. A week later, Rosa, on the advice of friends, consulted a burn specialist in a nearby city. He changed the treatment once again. Rosa's leg, while still painful, began to heal, and ten days later she felt she was almost completely recovered. She felt it was a wise move to have consulted the burn specialist who gave her such good care, and wished that the two previous doctors had done as well for her; she might have saved herself quite a bit of time and money, she figured.

Rosa's plight is not uncommon. The ability to judge good

medical care is difficult to come by for nonphysicians—and it sometimes appears difficult for physicians themselves to judge one another's performance. In Rosa's case, it would appear the third doctor gave good care and the other two didn't—but that's a surface judgment based on the fact that she got better. Would she have gotten better—perhaps within the same time period—had she continued to follow the advice of the first physician, or the second? Perhaps so, but Rosa will never know!

Good-quality care is sometimes measured by the outcome, but it is also measured by the process of care. Did the doctor do the right things within the limits of his knowledge, of medical knowledge in general, and of patient cooperation? Can the doctor be held accountable for more than this? There are no easy answers to these questions. Even the rare physician referred to as "a doctor's doctor," the person doctors themselves would rely on for medical advice, has his share of failures. Sometimes these are the result of an error on his part, but more often the result of a combination of circumstances over which he has no control. Even in these days of federally mandated review of the quality of medical care, doctors have a difficult time getting a handle on the meaning of the word "quality."

The dilemma faced by doctors in this area serves to point up the difficulty patients have in evaluating the quality of care they're getting from their own physicians. Following are some criteria which may help you get an indication.

1. *Have you selected your doctor wisely?*
   Review the criteria set forth in Chapters 2 and 3.
2. *Is your doctor keeping up in medicine?*
   Review the section on education, Chapter 3.
3. *Are the doctor, his staff, and his office clean and reasonably well organized?*
   Cleanliness and good organization in a medical practice do not necessarily imply high quality of care, but you can safely assume that a sloppy practice

with unkempt aides, a dirty office, and a dirt-under-the-fingernails doctor reflects a level of concern inconsistent with good-quality care.

4. *Do the doctor and his staff pay close attention to detail?*

The complexities of modern medical practice require this concentration. It's a good sign when the doctor asks probing questions, does a thorough check during the physical exam, and records his findings in your medical record before they escape his memory. It's also a good sign if the doctor's nurse or assistant takes time to explain how and why certain procedures are done.

5. *Does the doctor take time to listen?*

Remember that the doctor cannot make a proper diagnosis unless he listens carefully to your complaints, and to the answers to his questions. If you feel he isn't concentrating on you and you're only getting half an ear—and if this happens more than once or twice—then you have reason to be concerned about the quality of care that may result.

6. *Has the doctor made an effort to take a full profile of your health?*

Your primary physician should conduct a complete history and physical examination to give him baseline information needed to evaluate the state of your health and any subsequent illness. In some cases he may collect this information piecemeal, over a period of months. A specialist should have enough basic data to evaluate the condition he is diagnosing or treating. If, however, the doctor simply treats you for whatever ails you at the moment, he is not doing all he and you can do to safeguard your health and happiness.

7. *What is your doctor's attitude toward laboratory tests, X rays, etc.?*

Take heed if your doctor's attitude is at either

extreme—that is, if he goes overboard on the use of diagnostic tests, or if he shuns them like the plague. The sophisticated tests available to physicians today play a valuable role in diagnosis and in monitoring treatment for a number of diseases. In recent years, some physicians have become fascinated by the wealth of new laboratory tests available and tend to order an extensive battery of them when a small group might do as well. Or they have tended to hospitalize patients for a series of X rays and other examinations, when one or two such tests might have been performed on an outpatient basis with 95 percent coverage of the possibilities. On the other hand, some physicians of the old school have rebelled against what they consider over-reliance on tests by medical-center doctors, and have tended to rely almost completely on their own eyes and ears. Somewhere in between lies the rational course that is followed by physicians concerned about both the patient's well-being and his pocketbook.

8. *What is your doctor's attitude toward the use of medication?*

Good signs to look for are these: Before prescribing, the doctor checks on the drugs you are currently taking, whether another doctor has also prescribed for you, and whether you have any allergies to certain drugs such as penicillin or sulfa. He is cautious in his use of habit-forming drugs such as barbiturates, amphetamines, or tranquilizers, limiting the amount in each prescription and requiring his approval prior to repeated refills. He informs you of the name, strength, dosage, and timetable for taking the drug and has the druggist put this information on the label. He alerts you to possible side effects and what to do if they occur. Danger signs to watch for: The doctor who dispenses (sells) all the medications he prescribes (the doctor in a rural area is an exception). The doctor who routinely gives shots of penicillin, B-12, or other medications for almost any complaint. The doctor who prescribes by phone for a patient whom he does not know or has not seen in recent months.

9. *How carefully does he follow up?*

Good follow-up requires cooperation from the patient, but the doctor should explain carefully what is required and why, and have his office follow up at an appropriate time interval to insure compliance. Example of good practice: After diagnosing a urinary-tract infection, the doctor instructs the patient to take medication for ten days to two weeks and then return to his office with a urine specimen to be checked for absence of infection. The office calls the patient after three weeks if the patient has not reported in. Too often, the patient may feel better after three or four days of therapy, stop taking the drug, and forget about following up until the infection recurs with worse symptoms two or three months later. Clearly the patient has a responsibility —but so does the doctor.

10. *What is your doctor's attitude toward getting another opinion?*

Be wary of the doctor who resists the idea of having you get a second opinion, or who embarks on two or three quite different courses of treatment, one after the other, without a consultation.

11. *Are you satisfied that the doctor is giving you enough information about what he is doing?*

The quality of your care depends to a great extent upon your effective participation in it. You can't participate fully if you are in the dark about the diagnosis, the course of treatment, or where it is all heading. Ideally, the physician should review with you the key elements of your medical record and/or give you a copy of his diagnosis and of his treatment plan for you.

12. *Are you satisfied that the doctor knows what he is doing?*

Your confidence in the doctor is just as important as your participation in your care. If you feel that the doctor is floundering without seeking help, then it may be time for you to seek another opinion on your own.

13. *Are you getting better?*

The simplicity of this question suggests that it should come first. In reality, it's not the best criterion for judging the quality of care. For one thing, most diseases are self-limiting; that is, they will clear up or stop spreading by themselves given time, good health habits, and no complicating factors such as the coexistence of a chronic disease. This is not to say that the patient shouldn't see the doctor. The patient himself cannot judge whether or not he has a self-limiting disease, what the complications might be, or how much time may be required for the cure. The doctor's diagnostic and therapeutic skills not only deal with these questions, but can also relieve pain, reduce disability, and restore peace of mind. In some cases, however, the cure can be worse than the cold. Because of drug reaction, for example, it may take you longer to feel better than would have been the case without the drug. This is a risk that cannot be blamed entirely on the doctor, since the drug may work effectively 95 percent of the time. On the other side of the ledger, your failure to get better may be a reflection of the disease you have, or a result of your failure to follow instructions. Perhaps the least confusing response to this question is: If you aren't getting better, talk this over with your physician or get another opinion.

14. *What are your friends saying about the care you're getting?*

This is one way *not* to judge a doctor. The fact that cousin Sue had radio-iodine therapy for her enlarged thyroid gland doesn't prove your doctor wrong for recommending surgery if you have an enlarged gland. It's almost impossible for nonphysicians to compare symptoms and courses of treatment with any hope of being right. In fact, most doctors consulted on a curbstone basis would be extremely reluctant to evaluate the diagnostic or therapeutic decisions of a colleague who had actually examined the patient.

Even when two doctors of equal ability have the opportunity to investigate a patient's complaint in depth and prescribe treatment, their opinions may differ. Medicine is still an art, with vast territories open to legitimate debate and dispute. Technological advances in medicine are beginning to make it possible for doctors to agree upon minimal standards for the diagnosis and treatment of some diseases. But we are a long way from generally accepted standards of care that would cover the majority of patients seen in any medical office or hospital. However, given the same basic information about a sick patient, competent doctors in any part of the country are likely to arrive at a similar diagnosis and prescribe similar, though not necessarily identical, courses of treatment.

15

WHEN SHOULD YOU GET ANOTHER DOCTOR'S OPINION?

WHEN KEITH WILSON WAS THREE YEARS OLD, HIS PARENTS faced a difficult decision. Keith's pediatrician told them that their son would face serious loss of hearing as a result of chronic ear infections if he did not have surgery to drain the ears and to remove the adenoids. He referred Keith to an otolaryngologist for an evaluation and surgery. Even though he confirmed the pediatrician's recommendation, the parents were not satisfied. They sought still another opinion from a professor of ear diseases at a university center. His word was enough; when he agreed with the previous two opinions, Mr. and Mrs. Wilson immediately admitted Keith for the surgery, from which he recovered uneventfully with no further hearing impairment expected.

The Wilsons exercised good judgment by getting an additional opinion while at the same time satisfying themselves that they were doing everything that they could for Keith. When your health is at stake, or the health of someone in your family, you should be the one to make the final decision, based on the best advice you can get. The principles of medical ethics of the American Medical Association echo this concern for an additional opinion when appropriate: "A physician should seek consultation upon request; in doubtful or difficult cases; or whenever it appears that the quality of medical care may be enhanced thereby." Here are five basic situations in which you should seek another medical opinion:

1. *If your doctor recommends surgery.* The indications for surgery keep changing over the years, no matter what the condition. Medical-surgical controversies still exist over when to perform hysterectomies, mastectomies, cholecystectomies (for gallstones), herniorrhaphies (repair of hernia) and other procedures. When surgery is not deemed to be absolutely necessary for preservation of life and function, it is referred to as "elective surgery." Whether such surgery should be done is a matter of opinion by doctors and patients, and opinions change. For example, the rate of appendectomies and tonsillectomies appears to be going down, while the rate of hysterectomies is going up. In some parts of the country, back surgery is done three times as frequently as in other parts of the country. Very little surgery is completely unnecessary, but there may be serious questions as to whether the benefits of the surgery, in terms of quality of life and length of life, are worth the risks and the costs of the operation.

    Therefore it's wise to get more than one opinion when surgery is recommended. Find out what the potential benefits of the surgery will be, what the risks are, and what might happen if the surgery is not performed. Ask if alternative medical therapies are available and how they compare. In some cases, seek a second opinion from an internist, pediatrician, or family physician rather than from another surgeon. Use your primary physician as the source of referral to consultants.

2. *If your doctor makes a diagnosis of a potentially fatal or disabling disease.* Common sense should apply. If you have been told that you have a disease which is

going to kill you, certainly you have nothing to lose by getting another opinion. Doctors are not infallible, and there will be at least a small chance that the original diagnosis was not accurate. Or another doctor may be aware of a new therapy with which the first one was not acquainted. Obviously you owe it to yourself and to your family to get that opinion.

In one case a thirty-five-year-old father of a young family was dying of what had been diagnosed as a rare and untreatable form of cancer. Through a friend he was offered an opportunity to visit a reputable cancer hospital in another part of the country, which was experimenting with a new treatment for this type of cancer. Without making the trip, he allowed himself to be convinced by his own doctor that the experiment would fail and that they were doing all that was possible for him. Perhaps the new therapy would have indeed failed, but perhaps, too, he was ignoring the best interests of himself and his family in turning it down. I'm not suggesting that a person chase across the country or around the world seeking a miracle cure for an incurable disease, but another opinion from a leading physician or institution specializing in the disease is definitely advisable.

3. *If symptoms persist after a reasonable length of time under treatment.* Whether a disease is acute or chronic, there is usually some relief of symptoms that can be provided by the doctor—assuming that he is on the right track with his diagnosis. For example, he cannot cure a chronic disease such as diabetes or hypertension; but if he has correctly identified the nature and severity of the illness he can prescribe medications and other therapy that will alleviate such symptoms as fatigue, dizziness, itching, etc. If there is not noticeable relief after a two-to-three-month period—and you have told the doctor that you feel no better—then it's probably time to get another opinion.

Keep in mind, however, that some chronic diseases such as asthma, rheumatoid arthritis, and eczema are difficult to treat; in these instances you should not become dissatisfied if symptoms persist or recur with only a slight amount of relief from treatment. Even in these cases, for your own peace of mind you may want to seek another opinion after three to six months.

4. *If you feel that the doctor is not doing all he should.* You must have confidence in your doctor if his treatment is to be effective. Failing that confidence, you really will be well advised to seek another opinion, which hopefully will confirm the diagnosis and treatment of the first doctor.

If you have undergone surgery, for instance, it may seem to you that your recovery rate is much slower than it should be, and you may fear that a complication may have set in. If your surgeon's responses don't satisfy you, this is a time to seek another medical opinion. Or perhaps your pediatrician has said that your baby has a heart murmur, but it's nothing to worry about. If you're not sufficiently reassured, then by all means have another doctor examine the baby.

If you suspect that the recovery rate is not proceeding rapidly enough in spite of your doctor's assurances, seek other medical advice.

5. *If the diagnostic procedures or therapy advised appear complex, inappropriate, and/or very expensive.* Some doctors go overboard in their use of new technology in borderline situations. For example, one cancer specialist told me that occasionally a patient will relate that he or she was treated with an inappropriate and costly treatment modality for a certain condition, even when the patient had doubts. One patient had been given X-ray therapy for pain in her hip, with no evidence of malignancy.

The specialist added: "I was amazed that she would allow her doctor to do this, but indeed she did. She is an intelligent person and one who is usually discriminating about her medical care. I have also seen patients allow themselves to be subjected to rather formidable diagnostic procedures for questionable reasons." So, if you feel uneasy, by all means discuss your concerns and, if necessary, get a consultation.

Having decided that you want another opinion, how do you go about getting one?

The first step is to *talk openly with your own doctor about your concern.* Any doctor worth his salt should be willing to have his judgment confirmed by another physician, and should be willing to suggest the names of several specialists from whom you can make a choice. If he is repeatedly opposed to the idea of consultation, beware! Most physicians recognize that a consultant will either make them look good or save them a big mistake.

The simplest way to introduce the subject is to say something like this: "Would you mind if I saw another physician just to check out what you have told me? I think I owe it to myself and my family to be sure before going ahead."

Once having secured his agreement, even if grudgingly, let him recommend the doctor. If you have someone in mind, mention his name *after* your doctor has made his suggestions, and get his reaction. As a rule, you should ask the doctor's help in identifying the consultant who not only is best qualified medically to deal with the problem, but who also has the best rapport with your doctor and your personality.

This step can save a lot of time for both you and the consultant. Your own doctor will be in a position to help make the appointment with the consultant, to give him any background information he may need, and to get a report back from him quickly. Otherwise the consultant may repeat many of the diagnostic procedures and perhaps some of the therapy already attempted by your own physician. It will also prevent any misunderstanding on the consultant's part, so that he will not think you are coming to him as a regular patient.

Unless for some reason you are ready to change doctors, you should make it clear to your own doctor and to the consultant that you simply want a crosscheck in this particular case. Mention to both physicians that you would like a report by the consultant sent to your own doctor. Then make an appointment with your own doctor for a follow-up visit to review the report. Of course, you should also expect the consultant to give you a verbal report of his findings. However, it's not advisable to press him for a personal judgment on the ability of your own doctor. The consultant's report should speak for itself in terms of confirming or varying from your own doctor's opinion.

Suppose your own doctor is not willing to recommend a consultant? Then follow the advice for selecting a physician presented in Chapter 3. If possible, choose a man who has a subspecialty covering your particular illness.

When you are hospitalized with a serious disease and are being treated by a physician who is not a specialist in that specific disease, you usually have the protection of an automatic consultation. For example, most larger hospitals require consultations by a cardiologist in the case of a heart attack; a gastroenterologist must be consulted when gastrointestinal bleeding is present. If you are unsure about the rules for consultation in your hospital, do not hesitate to ask your doctor. A consultation by a qualified specialist may be a routine part of your care.

16

WHAT TO DO IF YOU'RE DISSATISFIED WITH YOUR DOCTOR

TED KERN, A TWENTY-YEAR-OLD COLLEGE BASEBALL PLAYER, was discovered to have a heart murmur on a routine college-sports physical exam. His parents asked him to come home to have their family doctor examine him in more detail and give them a full report. The family doctor referred Ted to a local hospital for a set of highly specialized tests and then Ted returned to college. A few days later, having heard nothing from the family doctor, Ted's mother called to find out the results. She was naturally anxious and pressed the doctor for information. He became annoyed, indicated that he didn't have time to deal with "hysterical mothers," and by his bluster covered up the fact that he had failed to follow up with the hospital to get the test results. A week later, he finally had his office assistant call back to report that a cardiologist had looked at the tests and felt there was nothing to worry about—unless Ted were a professional athlete. The Kerns felt that they had been treated cavalierly and still didn't really know what the heart murmur was all about. Their decision: change doctors.

The Kerns' annoyance was not unique. There are problem physicians as well as problem patients—and we seem to be more aware of them all the time. People have become more and more sophisticated and more critical about their medical care. Time was when patients were generally loyal to their physicians and reluctant to believe that the doctor might have made a mistake. He or she may have looked after the family for years and helped more than one member through a crisis. The fact remains that most people will now examine their doctor closely, and if he is not delivering the kind of care expected they will not hesitate to make a change.

If you are dissatisfied with your care, is it worthwhile talking with the doctor before making the change? The answer depends on the cause of your dissatisfaction. A study of all the complaints lodged against physician members of the Richmond, Virginia, Medical Society in 1973 showed that 40 percent felt the physician had charged an "excessive" fee; 35 percent complained that the doctor hadn't spent enough time with them, didn't return phone calls, or was out of town; and 31 percent felt that the doctor's treatment had failed to cure their problem and were unhappy about the poor results. Fee complaints are best discussed with the physician or his office right away. Sometimes these are simply poor record-keeping in the doctor's office. Lack of availability or a supposed poor result are also problems which are best discussed directly with the doctor. Chances are it's worth letting him know how you feel before making a change. Your opinion may be colored by ignorance or misinformation—or a failure of the doctor to communicate effectively—and a little frank discussion can help straighten it out.

If, on the other hand, before or after such a discussion, you feel that personality is the problem—as the Kerns did—then don't waste your time or the doctor's talking about it; find another doctor you like better. Patients have a right to expect that their physician will respond to them as individuals in a sympathetic manner. Patients also have a right to expect that the physician will develop a plan of action to deal as quickly as possible with the medical problem and will communicate in sufficient depth and at a time appropriate to the seriousness of the problem—as the patient sees it. Certainly, patients should not feel "put down" by either the physician or his staff personnel for being ill.

These personality characteristics and communication skills are extremely important. However, they're not the only evidence of competence or incompetence. An elderly physician in upper New York State had been found incompetent in his diagnostic and therapeutic abilities in the judgment of his medical colleagues; in his case, it took more than a year to revoke his medical license because so many loyal patients *defended* him on the basis of his character and sympathetic care.

Physicians are now taking more steps than ever before to deal effectively with the colleague who has been charged with incompetence. But progress is still slow, because defining competence is a difficult process. Most people will agree that competence is the combination of knowledge, skills, and behavior that results in good patient care. But breaking down that general definition into specifics causes physicians themselves, medical societies, lawyers, and courts all kinds of headaches—and costs the general public a great deal of money because of the rising incidence of malpractice suits. Even though doctors and hospitals pay the premiums, the costs of these premiums are passed back to the general public through increases in fees, charges, health insurance rates, and taxes.

The question of what is malpractice is still being hotly debated. There is a difference between a matter of medical opinion, a bad result, and negligence. The American Society of Internal Medicine has stated that "a malpractice action is justified when a patient suffers injury, disability, or death as result of an act of negligence by a physician." But the society also states that "unanticipated therapeutic outcome which follows appropriate medical care is not malpractice and should not result in a malpractice action." How can you tell how to proceed if you feel that your doctor has been incompetent or that you have had a bad result which you suspect may be due to his incompetence?

Here are four standards of care that in effect constitute legal obligations on the part of the physician toward his patient. A violation of any of these may well be grounds for a lawsuit. However, as you will see, there is room within the framework of these for the doctor to follow varying procedures and to come up with a poor result—without it being malpractice.

1. The physician must obtain the patient's informed consent before treating him. This means that the patient must understand the risks involved in a procedure at the time he agrees to it; but it doesn't mean that the physician must explain every remote possibility and every little detail, nor does it mean that he must get a signed consent form every time he treats a patient. With routine office procedures the patient can expect that the doctor will explain the nature of treatment; by the fact of the patient accepting the treatment the doctor has obtained the patient's "implied" consent. In a more unusual office procedure or in the hospital, the patient should understand exactly what the physician intends to perform, should understand that the doctor will use his judgment in meeting any unforeseen conditions, and should understand that the doctor hasn't guaranteed a cure. If surgery is to be performed, these points should be covered in a written form to be signed by the patient after the explanation is given.

A patient has a legitimate basis for action against a physician or hospital if he was simply asked to consent to "any or all" procedures that might be performed; if he was asked to sign a consent form by an admitting clerk without explanation; or if consent was obtained just prior to surgery while the patient was under sedation. If the patient is a child or mentally incompetent adult, and consent is not obtained from at least one responsible adult—even though the patient consents—there may be grounds for a lawsuit. In cases where informed consent is not properly obtained, the physician is technically open to a charge of assault and battery.

2. In treating a patient, the physician must exercise reasonable care and skill in accordance with accepted medical practice and within the limits of his competence. The key words here are "reasonable" and "accepted."

As an example of "reasonable," a physician who injured a patient because he mixed up two bottles containing phenol and glycerine might be said to have failed to exercise reasonable care, simply because he kept the bottles next to each other on a shelf and didn't look carefully enough before he selected the one to be used in treatment. He would therefore be considered guilty of negligence or malpractice. On the other hand, a surgeon who inadvertently perforated a patient's bowel during an abdominal operation might not be guilty of negligence if it could be shown that the accident occurred because the patient's bowel was in an abnormal position.

The question of what is an acceptable standard may be extremely difficult to establish in court. At one time a physician's treatment was judged solely on the basis of the standards of similarly qualified physicians in the same locality; but recently, with the availability of high-speed transportation and communications, almost any physician may be judged on national standards instead. This does not mean that the same level of care is expected of small-town general practitioners and medical-center specialists. Each has to be evaluated according to his peers . . . which also implies that the physician himself must recognize his own limits of competence. A small-town G.P., utilizing a new technique he had just read about in an orthopedic journal in an attempt to save a patient's bone-diseased foot, might well be guilty of malpractice if he failed and the foot had to be amputated. An orthopedic specialist, following the same procedure with the same poor results, would probably not be guilty of malpractice. The G.P. would have stepped beyond the bounds of his competence; the specialist would have been following a more advanced idea in his own particular field.

3. A physician must adequately supervise any aspect of a patient's medical care that he delegates to subordinates. It is customary for a doctor to delegate certain responsibilities, including parts of an examination, injections, and certain forms of treatment such as physical therapy, to a nurse or other allied health person. This is perfectly acceptable legally, as long as the physician assumes responsibility for training and supervising his help.

He leaves himself open for trouble, however, when he permits a nonprofessional—that is, a medical assistant without special training—to give injections. If a bad reaction occurs, the doctor will have a hard time proving that such an aide was adequately qualified. Incidentally, keep in mind that the doctor may be responsible for the negligence of nurses or aides in the hospital, even though they may not be in his employ; they may be considered to be under his supervision under certain circumstances.

4. Once a physician accepts a patient he must not abandon him or her. This means that the physician must continue to care for the patient until he or she no longer needs treatment, or until the patient leaves the doctor of his own volition, or until the doctor adequately notifies the patient that he is no longer responsible for his care.

Is the doctor legally bound to keep seeing the same patient over a long period of time? Only if he is treating the patient for the same condition (for example, diabetes or heart disease) over that period of time and has not notified the patient that he can no longer provide care. It would not be considered abandonment if a physician were to refuse his services to a patient whom he had treated six months previously for an entirely different condition—particularly if the physician's records showed that he had completed treatment for that earlier complaint.

Suppose a patient with a bleeding ulcer or other serious condition refuses to follow the doctor's advice to enter the hospital and demands to be treated at home. If the doctor refuses to continue treatment after making his preliminary diagnosis, is he guilty of abandoning the patient? Probably not, if he made every effort to convince the patient that satisfactory treatment, in his opinion, could be obtained only in the hospital. In effect, the doctor would be inviting failure by agreeing to the home treatment.

The physician is within his rights to dismiss a patient for other reasons: making unreasonable demands, consistently breaking appointments, or nonpayment of medical bills. If the patient is dismissed, however, the physician is obligated to inform him in writing and to allow reasonable time to find another physician. The original physician must be available for emergency care during this interim period.

If a physician goes out of town, or becomes ill, he has an obligation to provide coverage by a competent colleague for any patient under his continuing care. The name, address, and phone number of the covering physician should be made available through the doctor's office or an answering service.

What are the doctor's responsibilities in an emergency? If a physician stops at a roadside accident, he is expected to render reasonable care in accordance with his skills and within the existing circumstances. If he has nothing but bare hands and a handkerchief to work with, he cannot be expected to give the same kind of care that he would at his office or a hospital. Or, if he is a specialist in ear diseases, he cannot be expected to set a fractured kneecap. However, if he initiates treatment at the scene, he has the responsibility to make certain that another doctor will carry on where he leaves off. Because many doctors have been fearful of suits stemming from roadside aid, a majority of states have passed so-called "Good Samaritan" statutes exempting physicians from civil liability when they have given emergency care in good faith.

A physician who refuses to stop and render aid, or who refuses to come to the scene of an accident, may expose himself to public abuse and even criticism from some of his colleagues. But as long as he does not accept the responsibility for care, he is not exposing himself to legal recourse. This is true even if the emergency patient is taken to the doctor's office or to a private-hospital emergency room.

If the emergency case happens to be a patient of that doctor, however, the situation becomes cloudy. If it is a genuine emergency and the doctor refuses treatment, he may have a hard time proving that he was not guilty of abandonment. Similarly, if a physician is on call in a hospital emergency room and fails to give care after being called, he is liable for any bad results.

The patient who feels he has a grievance against his physician for any of the reasons stated here has three alternatives open to him. He can talk the matter over with his doctor. He can contact the local medical society. He can call his lawyer.

In most cases it's well to check out these alternatives in the order listed. By starting with the doctor himself, the patient may clarify what is possibly an honest misunderstanding. Sometimes a physician may be unaware of a poor result from his treatment, and will be only too ready to remedy it if given a chance. Beware, too, of jumping to conclusions and legal action if one doctor criticizes the treatment given by another. Review the situation with the first doctor and give him a chance to answer the criticism. Medical opinion does allow ample room for honest differences.

The second alternative is the medical society. Most large county and state medical societies today have grievance committees or malpractice arbitration committees to examine complaints against individual physicians. Frequently a patient will get support from such a committee if his complaint has reasonable basis in fact. The usual procedure is for the committee to hear both the patient's and the doctor's story. If a doctor refuses to appear before the committee, it may suggest that the patient pursue legal action. In any case, if the committee feels redress is in order, it may offer to provide witness service for the patient. It is no longer true that doctors universally cover up for one another's mistakes. Responsible members of the profession are often willing to stand up for a patient who has been treated negligently.

In more and more areas of the country, medical societies are now reaching out to deal with incompetent physicians in a positive manner, to try to improve their behavior. The Minnesota State Medical Association has been seeking to identify physicians needing help to overcome problems which result in substandard performance in practice. The Washington State Medical Association has set up a hot-line phone number, open twenty-four hours a day, which may be called by any patient, family member, or other physician, to report instances of apparent incompetence. A special committee will collect information on the physician in question, and if intervention is warranted, case managers—physicians from a distant area—are brought in to call upon the physician. They attempt to persuade him to seek help and they follow up to see if he responds. If the system fails, the original informant is notified and may choose to get redress through a disciplinary body of the medical society or of the state medical board.

If a patient's grievance persists after pursuing the above alternatives, then is the time to seek a lawyer. Use caution in selecting the lawyer, however. Not every attorney is capable of handling a negligence suit against a physician; this requires a knowledge of both negligence law and medical practice. Start by asking your personal attorney for a recommendation. Check to make sure that the man he suggests has had experience in representing plaintiffs in medical malpractice actions. Or call your nearest bar association and ask for their referral service. Most such cases are taken on a contingency basis, with the attorney charging his client a percentage of the settlement (ranging from 30 to 50 percent plus his own expenses).

For the most part, you can avoid the unpleasantness of taking a doctor to court by using your head early. If you begin to lose confidence in your physician, change doctors, or seek another opinion, which may restore your confidence in the first doctor. If your own doctor isn't available when you feel he's needed, bring up the question with him and if you still aren't satisfied, then seek another physician. Finally, make sure you understand just what the doctor is going to do before he does it. Raise your doubts and your questions then.

17

WHEN AND WHY TO GO
INTO THE HOSPITAL

ESTHER SMITH WAS SEVENTY-FIVE AND IN FAILING HEALTH, A widow who lived alone on a limited income. One day, while her regular doctor was on vacation, Esther began to suffer dizzy spells and blackouts. Her daughter, who lived close by, summoned a substitute physician to the house; he recommended immediate hospitalization for diagnostic tests. Six weeks later, Esther returned from the hospital to her home, a completely broken woman, failing not only in body but also in mind. The tests had shown a variety of chronic diseases, difficult to manage singly but almost impossible in combination. The hospital stay also resulted in Esther's disorientation, the beginnings of mental deterioration. She lingered several months at home, bedridden and barely able to recognize her daughter or other family members. Nursing care around the clock drained her already-meager resources to the breaking point. Her daughter later said, "I wish I had never put mother in the hospital, but had left her to die peacefully and comfortably at home."

Lila Bolt, a mother and homemaker in her early fifties, had twice had surgery for cancer: a radical mastectomy and a hysterectomy. She had undergone radiation therapy and chemotherapy, was bedridden periodically, and was in considerable pain. Her doctors felt there was indication that her cancer was spreading again, and urged her to enter the hospital for still another operation. Except for her husband's pressure, she would have declined, preferring to live out her few remaining months or years with her family without another painful operation. But she consented, entered the hospital, and underwent two extensive operations which removed many of her remaining glands. After a slow six-month recovery, Lila began to feel better than she had in years. She picked up the threads of her family and social life, and three years later appeared to have returned to a healthy, reasonably normal existence.

Should Mrs. Smith and Mrs. Bolt have entered the hospital when they did? For each, the costs of hospital care for the episodes described exceeded ten thousand dollars. With hindsight, Mrs. Smith might have been just as happy to stay at home, and the family and society would have been spared pain and expense. But Mrs. Bolt, almost miraculously, regained her life when it appeared lost.

Not every decision to hospitalize is as dramatic. But many are in this category, particularly nowadays when hospitals offer extremely sophisticated and high-cost technology, such as kidney dialysis and intensive respiratory care. At the same time that doctors are recommending more frequent use of these new technologies to save or prolong lives, other physicians are encouraging reductions in hospital stays for the traditional purposes, such as tonsillectomy, ulcer surgery, and infectious diseases. In some cases, physicians now believe they can treat certain diseases just as effectively at home as in the hospital. It has been traditional in the last thirty years to hospitalize patients with heart attacks. A recent study in England appears to indicate that certain heart-attack patients do just about as well being treated at home. But the evidence isn't conclusive yet.

In other cases, doctors recognize that some previous indications for surgery no longer are valid. It's uncommon, for instance, that a child needs his tonsils out these days; doctors used to remove them in order to prevent recurrent infections that now can be treated with antibiotics. The clear-cut cases still involve those in which surgery is definitely indicated, such as hip fractures, appendectomy, or cataract removal.

In addition to changing medical knowledge and concepts, the changing nature of the hospital itself causes patients and their doctors to reconsider the question of when to enter the hospital. The costs of hospital care have soared, and there is increasing pressure from health insurers, including the federal government, to monitor and reduce the incidence of unnecessary hospitalization. In New York State, for example, hospitals with a high number of Medicaid (or indigent) patients may have a team of state-paid doctors and nurses continually reviewing hospital admissions to determine whether or not the patient really belongs in the hospital. The purpose: to save dollars.

Some hospitals now have outpatient surgery departments, permitting a patient to come in early in the morning, have minor surgery, and be released the same day without spending the night. Even more hospitals have enlarged their emergency rooms and outpatient departments to provide routine as well as urgent care to ambulatory patients. Hospital administrators are under pressure to hold costs of care down while at the same time providing the newest types of care. Further, where there used to be a shortage of hospital beds, now in many areas of the country there are too many.

So doctors and patients have no easy time deciding when to use the hospital. Many cases appear to be routine decisions, but even these are changing. One study of factors leading to preventable hospital admissions showed that hospitalization could have been avoided for about half of a group of patients at Massachusetts General Hospital in Boston, had the course of the illness been modified appropriately at an earlier stage. In some cases, patients had delayed consulting a doctor; in many cases, doctors hadn't acted swiftly enough to prevent the illness from becoming severe enough to require hospital care.

This matter of prevention of hospitalization is important, not only because of the cost of hospitalization, but also because of the fact that perhaps about as many as one out of three hospital patients encounters a problem that he never would have had if he had not entered the hospital. These include a complication of surgery, an infection, a fall, an adverse reaction to medication, or a mistake in care on the part of a hospital employee.

Entering the hospital is a gamble, a gamble that may save your life or prolong it, but one that also carries certain risks. Among the questions you should ask your doctor are these:

1. What difference will it make if I do go to the hospital? Will it prolong my life—and by how much? Will it improve the quality of my life? In what way?
2. What are the specific risks I run by entering the hospital?
3. How can I avoid entering the hospital? Is there any course of treatment that might be an appropriate alternative on an outpatient basis? Is there an alternative form of care, such as a nursing home or a home health agency, available?
4. What will the economic and social impacts of my hospitalization be on me and my family? Will I become dependent on others for physical support?
5. Is there anything to be gained by waiting? Is there anything to be lost?

Don't hesitate to get a second opinion if in doubt, but remember to weigh both opinions carefully. A second opinion is often no better or worse than a first. Use your primary physician as a resource to discuss these questions and to help you reach a decision.

18

WHAT TO ASK YOUR DOCTOR— IN THE HOSPITAL

BURT WILLIAMS, A FORTY-YEAR-OLD PUBLISHING EXECUTIVE, was lying face down on the operating table, seeing only legs move back and forth in his range of vision and hearing cryptic comments from doctors and nurses around him. He had been taken to surgery about thirty minutes earlier to have a lipoma, or fatty tumor, removed from his shoulder. No one had spoken to him since rolling him from his room to the operating table. Finally, as he sensed the nearness of the surgeon's scalpel, he rose up on one arm, turned to the doctor, and asked whether he was going to be given an anesthetic. His surgeon barked back: "What's the matter with you? You sure have a lot of confidence in me!" With no further explanation, the surgeon proceeded with his work (which did include the injection of an anesthetic solution prior to removal of the tumor).

Burt Williams' experience is not unique. In hospitals across the country, patients reach a critical moment in their medical care without sufficient information, sometimes because they fail to ask the right questions at the right time— which is before being on the operating table—and sometimes because their physicians fail to provide the right information at the right time.

The problem is compounded because some patients are too intimidated by—or too trusting of—the health-care system to ask the questions in their minds, and because some physicians are so concerned about their own problems or egos that they fail to respond adequately to patients' questions, as was the case with Burt Williams' surgeon. Then, too, hospital care is often under the direction of a specialist who is not the patient's own primary physician. Information exchange is thus poorer in the hospital than in the doctor's office. The risks are higher, yet many patients just don't seek or receive the information they should have in order to make an informed decision.

In a roundtable discussion I moderated for *Patient Care* magazine a few years ago, I asked a panel of consumers and physicians these questions: "When you're hospitalized, how readily is information made available, not only to you but to your personal physician? Is he sufficiently informed to shoulder the ongoing responsibility to which we give so much lip service?"

Sallie Adams, a young consumer advocate, responded, "While I was a patient on and off for a year and a half in two Massachusetts hospitals, the process was one long fight for information. By virtue of that experience I came to my present point of view: What is practiced in hospitals is essentially veterinary medicine as far as informed consent is concerned. Neither I nor my personal physician—who's terrific—was kept adequately informed by hospital staffs. Thus I was submitting to care without granting informed consent and my G.P. was unable to carry continuing responsibility for my care.

"For example, the surgical residents [doctors in training] at one hospital made their rounds at six o'clock in the morning when a sleepy, medicated patient is unlikely to fire any questions. Whatever I did ask, the doctors took the attitude, 'There, there, don't you worry your pretty little head about it!' "

Obtaining adequate information from doctors in the hospital is essential to your own well-being, psychic as well as physical. Asking the right questions at the right time, and getting adequate answers, can help you avoid unnecessary surgery, can help you understand and accept the risks that go with hospital therapy, and can reduce the psychological impact of recovering from serious surgery or medical therapy. The 1976 edition of the Accreditation Manual for Hospitals, published by the Joint Commission on Accreditation of Hospitals, states that "the patient has the right to communicate with those responsible for his care, and to receive from them adequate information concerning the nature and extent of his medical problem, the planned course of treatment, and the prognosis." This statement relates to the doctrine of informed consent, the lack of which can form the basis for a medical malpractice suit.

Dr. Richard F. Gibbs, writing to physicians in the *Journal of Legal Medicine,* elaborates this doctrine to say that "every patient has a fundamental right to know and understand in a general way what is medically wrong; what the health-care provider plans to do about it; what the potential risks of treatment are; what alternative measures exist, along with their potential risks; and, finally, the probable outcome if only the most conservative or 'do-nothing' procedures are elected." Dr. Gibbs notes that a patient's failure to ask questions "or the trusting expression on his face, while indicative of confidence in the physician, should not be construed as implying full understanding of what was said."

Here are some guidelines that should be useful for asking questions and getting the answers about hospital care:

1. *Ask why the recommended treatment is necessary.* The patient in the bed next to Burt Williams was "scared to death" because his doctor had told him that he would probably need surgery to replace his pacemaker (an electrical device used to help maintain heart rate)—but he didn't know why. He didn't understand what was malfunctioning, since he felt generally all right, nor did he under-

stand why surgery would be necessary, but he was afraid to ask his doctor. Make sure that your doctor explains, in terms you understand, what the medical problem is and why the particular course of treatment, diagnostic test, or surgical procedure is necessary.

2. *Ask what the alternatives are.* There may be two or three methods of reaching a diagnosis or treating a disease. Another alternative may be to do nothing. (The results of "benign neglect" of a few diseases appear very little different from aggressive intervention with drugs or surgery.) Your doctor should explain to you what the alternatives are, and why he has recommended a particular course of action. Sometimes the weighting of the alternatives is a matter of which physician is responding to your question. A surgeon is more likely to look highly on surgical alternatives, an internist to favor medical alternatives. Put the same question to both your primary physician and your hospital specialist.

3. *Ask what the risks are.* For the management of almost all diseases that are treated in hospitals, some statistical probability tables have been developed on the frequency with which death and serious complications occur. In most hospitals, these data are available for the local hospital as well as nationally and regionally. (One common source of such statistics is the Commission on Professional and Hospital Activities, Ann Arbor, Michigan, which surveys more than 3,000 hospitals in the United States and Canada.) Ralph Berry, Ph.D., economics professor at Harvard, suggests that doctors should use probability distributions and decision-tree analysis of quantitative data along with qualitative judgments. "This was brought home when my son became a candidate for tonsillectomy," Dr. Berry told me. "He came through fine. But I have since been shocked to learn that mortality rates and adverse side effects from tonsillectomies—and surgery—are not trivial. When my next child becomes of operable age, I will insist that the doctor tell me what the probability distribution is of death and

adverse affects." You may not look for the precision of information Dr. Berry is seeking, but you do have a right to know what the risks are. You are the one person undergoing —or choosing for a loved one—that particular procedure or course of treatment, and you have a right to decide based on full information.

4. *Ask for a second opinion regarding a life-threatening procedure.* Sometimes the doctor's explanation makes sense, but the risks of what he is recommending seem very high. The view of another competent physician, preferably one *not* closely associated with your own physician, can be extremely helpful in arriving at a decision. In some states, Blue Cross and Blue Shield even pay for this additional opinion, particularly when surgery is involved. In the state of Illinois, for example, a subscriber to Blue Cross who has had surgery recommended can call a hot-line number and get the names of three consultants in the area. If, after a consultation, the second opinion concurs with the first, the patient has the first doctor proceed with the surgery (and Blue Cross pays all the bills for both opinions). In many areas of medical care, there is room for legitimate differences of opinion. When your life is at stake, it's worth getting the best *combined* advice possible. If the second opinion differs from the first, ask your family physician or internist to talk to both specialists and then help you to reach a decision.

5. *Ask for details of the recovery period.* The most common question is: "When will I be able to go home?" What's equally important is a detailed rundown on the effects of the surgery or other treatment. How long will you continue to tire easily? How long before you can get back to office work or housework, before you can resume playing golf or tennis, before you can drive your car again, before you can resume sex? How long will some pain or limitation of activity persist? Will exercise help or hurt? One useful trick here is to think about the activities that you've been carrying on in a typical week or month of your life in the past year.

Review these with your doctor to get some idea of how long it will be before you can resume that level of activity, and how to get there most quickly. Frequently your doctor doesn't know what you've been doing, and his response may not be geared to your experience unless you ask specifically.

6. *Ask about the emotional impact.* Most surgery does leave emotional as well as physical scars. It's well known that the loss of any body organ, such as a uterus, results in a grief reaction. Patients who have had heart surgery frequently undergo depressions after surgery. Most such psychic reactions to hospital procedures are of limited duration, but can be dealt with better if the patient is prepared. Otherwise anxiety over one's feelings can make the problem worse.

7. *Put your questions to the doctor who can answer them.* Dr. Gibbs says, "The person who is to provide the treatment should give the explanation and obtain the consent. This is not a ministerial function of nurses or other agents. It is the responsibility of each independent contractor in the health-care team to obtain his own consent, especially when risk is associated with an area under his specific direction and control." The doctor who is in charge of your care should be the one who answers your questions directly. If you have to turn to another doctor, a nurse, or a textbook for answers, chances are you will not get accurate responses.

8. *Put your questions and answers in writing.* Think through in advance the questions to which you want answers, discuss these with a close relative, and then commit them to paper. A hospital procedure is an important event in your life; it's worth the time to prepare your questions so that you make sure to cover everything. If the doctor appears rushed, make sure that he sets aside the time for another visit before you give your consent to proceed. Otherwise, like Burt Williams, you may have to put your question while on the operating table—and by that time your options are quite limited! If possible, write down the doctor's response to your questions and his explanations, or have a relative present to take notes. (The doctor should also be noting in his own

record what he has said.) This will make a useful document for later reference. In fact, a recent study by Dr. George Robinson, a professor of surgery in New York, showed that many of his open-heart-surgery patients did not remember the content of preoperative informed-consent conversations. In general, patients could recall only about 20 percent of what had been discussed before surgery. That's about what most of us remember from any conversation or even from a good sermon. And in the hospital, anxiety often blocks the ability to hear and remember. All the more reason to record the information so that it can be reread, rather than simply committed to memory.

19

HOW TO CHOOSE A HOSPITAL

LILLIAN LOOMIS WAS CONCERNED THAT HER SISTER, WHO WAS in the intensive-care unit of Community General Hospital, was not improving. Lillian called her own cardiologist, in whom she had a great deal of confidence, requesting that he take over the management of her sister's care. But the cardiologist could not do so. He had his office in a suburb only five miles away, but he did not have hospital privileges at Community General Hospital. He could have visited Lillian's sister, but he could not have assumed responsibility for her care in Community General unless he had been admitted to the hospital staff and had specific privileges to care for patients in the intensive-care unit.

Because of these limitations, your choice of a hospital is usually limited—to the hospitals in which your doctor has privileges. If you want to continue under his care while hospitalized, you must be admitted to one of these hospitals, and sometimes it is just one hospital. Of course, you could begin by choosing a hospital and then select a doctor on the staff, but in most cases you'll feel more reassured starting with a doctor you know and trust.

Given this restriction on choice, there are some important considerations that should be checked out by you or your family before entering a hospital:

1. *Is the hospital accredited?*

About forty-eight hundred of the seven thousand acute-care general hospitals in the country are accredited by the Joint Commission on Accreditation of Hospitals, a nonprofit organization originally formed by the American College of Physicians, the American College of Surgeons, the American Hospital Association, and the American Medical Association. The commission sets optimal rather than minimal standards for hospital care, covering:

Patients' rights
Policies
Quality of professional services
Building and grounds safety
Functional safety and sanitation
Infection control
Anesthesia services
Dietetic services
Emergency services
Governing body and management
Hospital-based home care
Medical-record services
Medical staff
Nuclear-medicine services
Nursing services
Outpatient services
Pathology services
Pharmaceutical services
Physical-medicine services
Professional library services
Radiology services
Respiratory-care units
Social services
Special-care units

Every year thirty-five survey teams review almost three thousand hospitals, assessing performance, recommending changes, and sometimes recommending that the Joint Commission revoke accreditation or put the hospital on one-year probation because standards are not met. (Normally, accreditation is for two years.) Nowadays revocation of accreditation is costly, because it may mean that a hospital will lose the right to collect Medicare and Medicaid payments for patients covered under those government health-payment programs, so most hospitals really make an effort to meet the accreditation standards and remedy any defects rapidly.

Accredited hospitals represent about 85 percent of all hospital beds; many small hospitals, particularly those under twenty-five beds, are not accredited. Those given full accreditation usually display their certificates in the lobby. If you don't see one, ask the hospital administration or check with the Commission, 875 North Michigan Avenue, Chicago, Illinois 60611. If a hospital is unaccredited, check to determine if it is approved for participation in Medicare and Medicaid programs. Standards for this are usually set by the state and may or may not be at the level of the Commission's standards.

2. *Is it a general or a special hospital?*

Most of the time you're better off in a general hospital rendering acute care; occasionally, you may find that a special hospital has specific services that you would not find elsewhere. For example, cancer patients might get the most up-to-date treatment at a major cancer center such as Memorial Hospital in New York City; M. D. Anderson Hospital in Houston, Texas; or Roswell Park Memorial Hospital in Buffalo, New York. Or a child with severe asthma might be better off at National Jewish Hospital in Denver, Colorado. In some large cities, special hospitals are maintained for children's diseases, obstetrics and gynecology, and chronic diseases in the elderly. Specialized mental hospitals are also widely available. A general hospital usually offers a complete range of services, with sections for pediatrics, internal medicine, obstetrics, and surgery. If the general hospital is a large university hospital, its sections may be divided further to include specialties such as ophthalmology, cardiology, gastroenterology, etc. The quality of care in any section of a university hospital may well be equivalent to that rendered in a special hospital, depending upon the physicians who are on the staff. Rural hospitals tend to be staffed by primary physicians (family physicians, plus some general internists, pediatricians, obstetricians and general surgeons). Specialized care is not likely to be available except by transfer to a larger urban hospital.

3. *Is it a teaching hospital?* A teaching hospital is one that has an approved program for teaching resident physicians. At the top of the ladder of teaching hospitals are the university hospitals, which form the bulwark of the clinical-training program for the nation's medical schools. The medical-school faculty provides most of the staff for the university hospital, and most patients are either referred there by local doctors or come in as indigent clinic patients. Another approach is the university-affiliated teaching hospital. This will usually be community-owned, but have one or more special teaching programs operated in cooperation with a medical school. Next is the community hospital having an approved residency program in at least two of the major specialties—family practice, internal medicine, surgery, obstetrics and gynecology, and pediatrics. There are about four hundred hospitals in the Council of Teaching Hospitals, the organization representing the major university-affiliated hospitals; they are generally located in large cities.

There is considerable debate over whether, given the choice, you should choose a teaching over a nonteaching hospital. If you are seriously ill, the answer is clear: you should be in a teaching hospital where specialized care and facilities are much more readily available. Some physicians would argue that *any* patient is better off in a teaching hospital, because the latest equipment and the best-trained physicians are available there. On the other hand, even some top men on medical-school faculties will tell you that the teaching hospital is no place to be sick—unless you are seriously sick. There is often a cold, impersonal atmosphere;

the patient is subjected to pawing and prodding by a string of residents and student nurses. The length of stay may turn out to be longer and the risk of infection higher. It must be remembered that in most teaching hospitals the primary goal is teaching, the secondary goal is patient care. Sometimes research comes ahead of patient care, too.

4. *How many beds does the hospital have?* Most university hospitals have between 500 and 1,000 beds, with many special sections. Most other teaching hospitals have 250 beds or more. As a rule, the quality of medical care is likely to be better in a hospital of 100 beds or more than in a smaller hospital. The larger one is likely to have more specialists on the staff, more special units such as coronary-care and intensive-care units, and more special equipment on hand to deal with emergencies. In many small rural hospitals it may be difficult to find any physician present in the hospital if an emergency comes up. The on-call physician may take ten to fifteen minutes to arrive. However, there are some small (25- to 50-bed) hospitals which offer better-than-average care. Marks of excellence include accreditation, the presence of one or more specialists on the staff, facilities for intensive care and coronary care, and nurses well trained in these special procedures and available in adequate numbers.

5. *Who operates the hospital?* Aside from university hospitals, most are set up as community, nonprofit corporations with a lay board of trustees and a constant need for public support. Some today are operated by religious groups. Finally, there are privately owned (for profit) hospitals, usually now operated by publicly held corporations, though in some cases run by physicians. Regardless of ownership, a hospital can gain accreditation. Investor-owned chains have rapidly purchased or built new hospitals in the past ten years; 31 multiple-facility corporations own most of the 1,000 for-profit hospitals in the country, and many of these corporations also have contracts to manage religious, county,

or community hospitals. At one time, for-profit hospitals tended not to offer as good care as nonprofit hospitals; that appears to be no longer true. The for-profit hospitals may offer fewer special services, but they frequently try harder to please both patients and doctors, in order to remain profitable.

As mentioned earlier, your doctor is usually the governing factor in your choice of a hospital. In many communities today, a physician generally narrows his work to one hospital because it is more convenient to have all of his patients in one hospital, and he has a better chance of getting a bed there when he needs it. The favored hospital also may grant him more extensive privileges than the others.

By privileges we mean that the doctor is permitted to treat certain types of patients and perform certain procedures in accordance with his training and demonstrated competence. Once licensed, a physician is legally permitted to perform a full range of medical and surgical services. In practice, he is governed to a large extent by his hospital privileges. Technically he applies to the hospital to perform those services which he feels he is capable of rendering, for example, general medicine, obstetrics, and minor surgery (tonsillectomy, hernia repair, etc.). A committee of the hospital medical staff will examine his record and determine whether or not to grant him the privileges he requests. Sometimes they will be granted on a probationary basis until his work has been observed for a period of six months to a year. In some areas, particularly in city hospitals, family physicians may be permitted an extremely limited range of privileges, usually excluding surgery. In rural hospitals, family doctors may be permitted to do major surgery; in fact, they will probably comprise the entire medical staff.

If your doctor has limited privileges and wishes to admit you to a hospital for a procedure he is not permitted to do, he will usually call in a consultant on the same hospital staff. This way you will have the benefit of your own doctor's continuing care and overall management, plus the help of the specialist. This is more common in the East than in the West.

Suppose you need hospital care and find that your doctor does not have privileges at a hospital that is most convenient to you, or one that offers special care of a type you desire. Your best bet is to discuss this problem openly with him. If it is simply a matter of convenience, and you have considerable confidence in your doctor, you are probably wiser to stay with his choice of a hospital. In other situations you can ask for a referral to a physician on the staff at the institution you prefer. Give serious weight to his opinion of the hospital; remember, doctors spend a good part of every day within those institutional walls—and your other sources of information may be people who have been in a hospital bed for only a few days or weeks of their entire lives.

Warning signs that may indicate a below-par hospital: financial problems or internal disputes reported by the local media, such as strife between the hospital administration and the doctors . . . strikes or unrest by hospital employees . . . a hodgepodge appearance as you walk through the hospital or signs of disorder . . . doctors on the staff who have had disciplinary action taken against them by the state licensing board or state medical society.

20

HOW TO EVALUATE
HOSPITAL CARE

TECHNOLOGY AND TEAMWORK ARE SAVING LIVES IN THE HOS-
pital, but sometimes at the expense of the personal contact
and compassion so necessary to good-quality care. Three
illustrations make the point:

Myrna Bergstrom, eighty-five, broke her hip. She was
taken to a medical-school hospital in the late evening by
ambulance. Her seventy-seven-year-old sister, who accompanied her to the hospital, wandered through basement corridors alone for an hour trying to find the office to which she
was told she must go in order to sign the necessary admitting
papers. Then she could not find her way back to the bedside.
Her pleas for help were brushed off by hospital personnel
who were "too busy" to guide her. Experts in medical care
might say this was not a true problem in the quality of care.
But to her and her sister, it was.

David Smith, age twenty, smashed through the windshield
of his car in a head-on collision. His parents waited outside
the suburban-hospital emergency room for an hour and a
half, during which the only communication was: "The
doctor is with him now, and will see you in a few moments."
The emergency-room personnel were busy giving care, but
not to the worried family.

Arthur Riley, age eighty-one, had been admitted to the coronary-care unit with an acute myocardial infarction. On the third day, as his wife was seated at his bedside, he grimaced in pain and the heartbeat recorded on the monitor over his head fluctuated wildly. Nurses and doctors rushed into the room, bodily removed the almost hysterical wife, and went to work to try to save Arthur. Three hours later he died, after a major arrhythmia (heartbeat irregularity). During that time his wife was not permitted to see him again, nor was she given any indication of his condition. In answer to her repeated frantic inquiries, she was told at various times: "He's resting now; you mustn't disturb him." "The doctors are with him, you can't disturb them." "Please leave us alone. We'll let you know when there's anything to report." And finally, from the cardiologist in charge of the unit: "We're sorry. He's gone. We did everything we could." Did they? Perhaps there was no question about the quality of the coronary care. But what about the quality of compassion?

Evaluating the quality of care in a hospital is a difficult task, even for professionals. But patients and their families can monitor certain factors in the way a hospital is run. Unfortunately, the time of hospitalization isn't the time to evaluate the hospital. Little can be done at that point, and complaints may only bring about emergency remedial action. The time to find out about the hospitals in your community is prior to hospitalization. This can be done through discussions with your doctor, with the hospital administrator, with the hospital public relations office, or with a member of the hospital Board of Trustees, most of whom are leading lay-persons in the community. Here are the points to check:

1. *The quality of medical care.* Regular evaluation of the quality of medical care is now a requirement by the Joint Commission on Accreditation of Hospitals (see Chapter 19) and by the federal government, through Professional Standards Review Organizations (PSROs). PSROs were set up in 1972 by Congress in order to monitor the appropriate-

ness of services and the quality of those services provided to patients covered by Medicare, Medicaid, and maternal/child programs of federal health insurance. Both the Joint Commission and PSROs require that hospitals regularly conduct audits of the care that has been rendered. Once problems in care have been identified, corrective-action programs are supposed to be set up among physicians, nurses, and other personnel. Sometimes these audits are conducted in order to whitewash the staff, but frequently they do in fact uncover problems that can be remedied through education, through changes of medical, nursing, or administrative procedure, or occasionally through disciplinary action.

Another method of monitoring the quality of medical care is through the credentials committee of the medical staff. This is the committee which reviews and recommends to the Board of Trustees of the hospital the credentials of each member of the medical staff and his or her requests for privileges to care for patients. If the credentials or other appropriate committee is performing its job properly, it should be examining the work done by each physician in accordance with his or her privileges, whether they be medical, surgical, obstetrical, or pediatric. In some cases, physicians may be put on probationary status and be required to seek consultation to handle more difficult problems in patient care. The stickiest area of monitoring quality is what to do about the elderly physician who is beloved by his colleagues and his patients, but whose advancing years have impaired his physical and mental skills. Too often a hospital credentials committee does not have the guts to reduce or eliminate the privileges of such doctors until the bad results begin to pile up.

A third element in monitoring quality of medical care is related to the special equipment and services a hospital has for handling diagnostic and treatment procedures, and the frequency with which those procedures are conducted. In general, except for rural areas, a hospital that has fewer than three hundred to four hundred deliveries a year probably should not be providing an obstetrical service. A hospital that has less than one open-heart operation a week probably should not be equipped for open-heart surgery. With a low frequency of such procedures, it's difficult to keep a trained staff and to afford all the equipment that's necessary for dealing with the unexpected complication.

2. *Quality of coordinated care.* Most patients need a primary physician to coordinate the care of specialists and subspecialists in the hospital, some of whom wouldn't recognize a patient by name or face without a view of the patient's abdominal incision. For example, if you are in a teaching hospital with a back problem, your attending physicians may include your family doctor, a neurosurgeon, a radiologist, and perhaps two or three resident physicians in medicine and surgery. Unless your family doctor coordinates the recommendations and actions of each team member, you may be subject to duplicate tests, contradictory treatments, and even omitted procedures, because each doctor thought another had done the job.

Similarly, you should have a primary nurse coordinating your nursing care. Many hospitals today have their nursing services organized so that for a group of eight patients, one nurse serves as the primary nurse, talking with each patient and family, arranging a nursing-care plan, and ensuring that it is carried out by the other nurses on duty in that section. The primary nurse becomes a liaison between the patient and the doctor and other personnel in the hospital in regard to clinical care.

Another type of coordinating person—on a nonclinical level—is the patient representative, or patient advocate. The patient representative's primary assignment is to serve as the liaison between patients and the institution as a whole, and between the institution and the community it serves. She enables patients and families to obtain solutions to problems by acting in their behalf with the hospital administrator or with any department or service. She listens to compliments as well as complaints, ascertains the feelings of patients and their families, assists in interpreting hospital bills and health insurance information, makes appointments with social workers or other community-agency people, assists patients in obtaining needed medical-record information, and even helps find lost or stolen articles.

3. *Quality of tender loving care.* Coordinated care is a prerequisite to tender loving care. Without a doctor, nurse, and/or patient representative providing an onging relationship, it's difficult for a patient to feel cared for in the highly specialized network that comprises today's hospital. Yet it's at just this point in life—when seriously ill—that caring becomes extremely important.

Hospitals today are staffed by a variety of personnel, including registered nurses, practical nurses, student nurses, nurses' aides, orderlies, ward clerks, and volunteers. Theoretically, the quality of bedside care would be highest if it were all rendered by R.N.'s. But the nursing shortage has forced most hospitals to keep R.N.'s in supervisory responsibilities and tasks calling for highly specialized training: giving injections, starting intravenous medications, etc. So if a non-R.N. shows up to change the bed, give a bath or enema, take a temperature, or give an oral medication, don't be disturbed. These functions can be adequately handled by nonprofessionals under supervision.

What should you look for in evaluating bedside care? First, does someone come within a minute or two, or respond by intercom, when you ring the call bell? Delays in answering a patient's call are an indication of inadequate staffing. (But don't wait until the last minute to call! Anticipate your need for a bedpan or medication.) Second, if you have a complaint, does the nurse call the doctor if she can't deal with it herself? As indicated above, the doctor has responsibility for most elements of your care. He should be informed if you have a change in your physical condition, if you are concerned about your medication or diet, if you want to know whether you can go into the bathroom or eat your dinner in a chair. Third, does a nurse check you periodically whether or not you have called? This is particularly important for a patient under sedation, or an older person who may not be familiar with his surroundings.

When is a private-duty nurse advisable? As a rule, your physician can advise you on this, and may even order one or more if the severity of the case warrants, and if a hospital intensive-care unit is not available. If there is any question about the adequacy of the nursing staff to deal with the questions just raised, then a private-duty nurse is probably good insurance for the first day or two following surgery, or during intensive medical procedures. This is particularly true when the patient is in a private room. The duty nurse is not as likely to check a private room as often as she will a room with multiple patients.

Tender loving care also implies a concern on the part of the hospital staff for the patient's family. Are there convenient places where family members can wait while the patient is under special care, and is there someone specifically delegated to keep the family informed of what is happening? This may not be a nurse, but may be an aide or volunteer who reassures the family, gives them periodic bulletins from the doctors and assists in moments of crisis. Unfortunately, few hospitals have provided this kind of special assistant. But more hospitals are permitting family members to stay with patients, recognizing the value of emotional and sometimes physical support during hospitalization. Fortunately, too, more hospitals are permitting parents to stay with sick children, and some hospitals provide sleeping accommodations in or near the child's room. (Sometimes, unfortunately, nurses and resident physicians have trouble handling the closeness of the family, because they feel uncomfortable when someone watches their activities.)

4. *Food and housekeeping service.* This area of hospital care probably causes more complaints than any other, perhaps because most people have a basis for comparison—and, by comparison, most hospitals aren't in a class with luxury hotels; but then they weren't meant to be.

Nevertheless, in a well-run hospital today, you should expect well-planned menus with a variety of items to choose from, and well-prepared food attractively served hot or cold —not lukewarm. If you are on a special diet, perhaps salt-free, you may, of course, find the food unappetizing, no matter how well prepared! Some hospitals serve extra meals in the room (at extra cost) to a visitor from the immediate family; some even include wine with the dinner. Touches like these can make a hospital stay more pleasant.

Housekeeping services are a different story. Here you have a right to expect the utmost in cleanliness, and a high degree of comfort. Floors, bathrooms, window ledges, etc., should be cleaned daily to reduce the risk of contamination and infection. Utensils such as water pitchers, bedpans, and trays should be cleansed regularly and changed from day to day. If you are a relative and have an opportunity to inspect hospital areas outside of the room, take a look into storerooms, closets, and the space behind emergency-exit doors. If these are kept immaculate, the rest of the hospital is likely to be.

5. *Physical plant.* The trouble with most hospitals today is that they were outmoded before they were built. Medical progress moves so rapidly that it is impossible to anticipate services and facilities that will be needed within a year. At a recent meeting of hospital consultants, one university authority suggested, "It would be ideal if there were some way that we could build a disposable hospital with a life-span of five years instead of fifty."

There are some trends in hospital planning worth noting, not so much because you can fault your hospital for lack of these facilities, but because you may be able to support a program incorporating them. A hospital should be part of a health-care center including a doctors' office building, social services, an extensive emergency service, and home health and rehabilitation agencies.

6. *Financial status.* A poorly financed hospital cannot maintain adequate personnel nor keep abreast of new de-

velopments in equipment and facilities. Some hospitals have been on the verge of bankruptcy—or in it—because they overextended themselves in major expansion efforts without adequate funding. Nonprofit hospitals should have a financial statement available on request.

Finally, find out if your hospital has adopted the patient's bill of rights (see below) recommended by the American Hospital Association, or a similar bill of rights. Recognizing that a hospital has many functions to perform, including teaching and research, the American Hospital Association states that "all these activities must be conducted with an overriding concern for the patient, and, above all, the recognition of his dignity as a human being." In these days of increasing depersonalization and institutionalization of patient care, more hospitals should adhere to the spirit as well as the letter of the patient's bill of rights.

A PATIENT'S BILL OF RIGHTS

Statement by the Board of Trustees,
American Hospital Association

1.   The patient has the right to considerate and respectful care.

2.   The patient has the right to obtain from his physician complete current information concerning his diagnosis, treatment, and prognosis in terms the patient can be reasonably expected to understand. When it is not medically advisable to give such information to the patient, the information should be made available to an appropriate person in his behalf. He has the right to know by name the physician responsible for coordinating his care.

3.   The patient has the right to receive from his physician information necessary to give informed consent prior to the start of any procedure and/or treatment. Except in emergencies, such information for informed consent should include but not necessarily be limited to the specific procedure and/or treatment, the medically significant risks involved, and the probable duration of incapacitation. Where medically significant alternatives for care or treatment exist, or when the patient requests information con-

cerning medical alternatives, the patient has the right to such information. The patient also has the right to know the name of the person responsible for the procedures and/or treatment.

4.   The patient has the right to refuse treatment to the extent permitted by law, and to be informed of the medical consequences of his action.

5.   The patient has the right to every consideration of his privacy concerning his own medical care program. Case discussion, consultation, examination, and treatment are confidential and should be conducted discreetly. Those not involved in his care must have the permission of the patient to be present.

6.   The patient has the right to expect that all communications and records pertaining to his care should be treated as confidential.

7.   The patient has the right to expect that within its capacity a hospital must make reasonable response to the request of a patient for services. The hospital must provide evaluation, service, and/or referral as indicated by the urgency of the case. When medically permissible a patient may be transferred to another facility only after he has received complete information and explanation concerning the needs for and alternatives to such a transfer. The institution to which the patient is to be transferred must first have accepted the patient for transfer.

8.   The patient has the right to obtain information as to any relationship of his hospital to other health care and educational institutions insofar as his care is concerned. The patient has the right to obtain information as to the existence of any professional relationships among individuals, by name, who are treating him.

9.   The patient has the right to be advised if the hospital proposes to engage in or perform human experimentation affecting his care or treatment. The patient has the right to refuse to participate in such research projects.

10.   The patient has the right to expect reasonable continuity of care. He has the right to know in advance what appointment times and physicians are available and where. The patient has the right to expect that the hospital will provide a mechanism whereby he is informed by his physician or a delegate of the

physician of the patient's continuing health care requirements following discharge.

11. The patient has the right to examine and receive an explanation of his bill regardless of source of payment.

12. The patient has the right to know what hospital rules and regulations apply to his conduct as a patient.

21

WHICH TYPE OF LONG-TERM CARE IS BEST?

WHEN HENRY HOWELL CAME HOME, HIS SEVENTY-THREE-year-old wife rejoiced. It had been six months since Henry's stroke; he had spent almost two months in the hospital and the balance of the time in a nursing home, where he had received a high degree of skilled nursing care. In spite of Martha Howell's bad back, she wanted to care for Henry at home without any help. The nursing-home administrator was worried when she heard this, so she sent a record of the case to a nearby home health agency, recommending follow-up by a visiting nurse. But Martha refused to admit the nurse to the house. Martha's daughter was contacted, and convinced her mother that the nurse would really help. When the nurse arrived, however, more problems arose: she felt that Henry really needed to be in a lower-level nursing home where he could get continuing care. Martha again rebelled. The nurse patiently taught her how to help Henry without hurting her back and assigned a home health aide to do the more exhausting chores of patient care. After two weeks, Martha realized that, much as she wanted Henry home, she physically was not able to give him the twenty-four-hour care he needed; she finally accepted the idea of a transfer to the nursing home.

The complex, agonizing dilemma of the Howells is becoming increasingly common in our society, in which some 40 percent of Americans have one or more chronic illnesses, and four out of five people over sixty-five have at least one chronic condition. More than half of these suffer varying degrees of disability. Who should care for them, and in what way?

In years past, families took care of their own ill and elderly, but in today's mobile society the task has become almost impossible. Family members may live hundreds or even thousands of miles apart. Houses are smaller and are seldom planned to accommodate three generations. An increasing number of women hold jobs. Children become accustomed to leading their own lives without day-to-day consideration for grandparents. In today's youth-oriented culture, there is an expectancy among the younger generations that they will live their own lives without the burden of responsibility for aging relatives. There are less guilt feelings about individual failure to carry this burden, because third parties—health-insurance companies and government programs such as Medicare and Medicaid—pay the lion's share of our health-care bills.

These changes in the family structure and in health-care financing have led to the development of a sophisticated range of long-term-care services. These consist of extended-care facilities, skilled nursing facilities, resident-care facilities, foster homes, home health-care programs, and day-care centers. In this chapter you will find each type of special care defined, the criteria for determining which type to use, and tips on how to learn which facilities are available in your area.

1. *Extended-care facilities.*

An extended-care facility is an establishment with an organized medical staff, and with continuous professional nursing service. It provides relatively short-term, comprehensive in-patient care, usually following a hospital stay, when a patient no longer needs the complete range of hospital services. It may also serve convalescent patients who are not in an acute episode of illness, but who have a variety of medical conditions needing skilled care.

Extended-care facilities are relatively recent intermediate steps between hospitals and nursing homes. Most frequently they are attached to hospitals, so that a patient may simply be moved from one wing to another. The cost of extended care may be one third to one half that of a hospital bed, because certain expensive services such as operating rooms and intensive-care units do not have to be carried by the extended-care facility. Nursing supervision is available, but not to the extent that it is in acute care.

Which patients are candidates for an extended-care unit?

(a) The patient who has had a coronary and is recuperating uneventfully after a two-week stay in the hospital.

(b) The patient who has undergone major surgery and has recovered to the point of being able to feed himself, move about his own room, and be on chiefly oral medications.

(c) The patient with a chronic illness such as diabetes or hypertension who has had a flareup of the disease and requires rest with careful medical supervision.

In these and other situations, the decision to use an extended-care facility rather than the hospital should be in the doctor's hands. It's clear from the examples given that there is often just a shade of difference in the level of care needed.

Many hospitals of two hundred beds or more have put in extended-care facilities in an effort to free regular hospital beds for acutely ill patients. In some cases a nursing home may have brought its level of care up to qualifications set forth by the Joint Commission on Accreditation of Hospitals, or by Medicare. If you are interested in determining whether or not your community has an extended-care facility, ask your doctor or hospital administrator.

2. *Nursing-care facilities.*

These are long-term skilled-care establishments having a

medical staff and continuous nursing service under the direction of professional nurses, but they are usually a step down from the extended-care facility. The level of medical and nursing supervision is less intensive, though still well above that of a home for the aging or a resident-care facility. Which patients are candidates for nursing-care facilities?

(a) The patient who is recuperating from a stroke, or from a fractured hip.

(b) The patient who requires frequent changes of dressings as a result of surgery or a serious skin condition.

(c) The patient who is dying of cancer or another fatal illness. (Also consider a hospice inpatient program or home-care program, described in Chapter 12.)

(d) The patient with severe disease of the muscles or joints, such as arthritis or multiple sclerosis.

(e) The patient with severe mental or nervous diseases, such as cerebral arteriosclerosis or Parkinsonism, which result in confusion.

A skilled-nursing-care facility—or nursing home—is designed to provide continuous medical care for any patient who needs it, but it should not be used as a dumping ground for every elderly or chronically ill person who is unable to care for himself at home.

3. *Residential-care facilities.*

A residential-care facility is an establishment providing safe, hygienic, sheltered living for people not capable of—or not desiring—fully independent living. It offers regular but not continuous medical and nursing services, and usually offers continuous supportive services such as food, a social program, and occupational or recreational therapy. In many cases, a residential-care facility will offer programs to assist a person in relearning the activities of daily living: that is, feeding, dressing, and grooming. At the upper level of residential care are nursing homes providing what is called custodial or protective care, and homes for the aging providing a full range of housekeeping, food, and social services. At the lower level are retirement villages or apartments, which are geared primarily for semi-independent living while providing some shared services.

Which persons are candidates for residential-care facilities?

(a)   The elderly couple who can no longer physically or financially run their own home.

(b)   The partially disabled person who no longer needs continuous medical care, but who cannot be completely self-sufficient.

(c)   The single elderly person who occasionally has episodes of confusion, depression, or anxiety.

(d)   The elderly relative who doesn't want to be alone, but at the same time does not want to live with his or her children.

In many cases, an elderly person will make the decision for himself or herself about a move to a residential-care facility. It may be precipitated by the death of a husband or wife, financial considerations, injury, or illness. When one of these precipitating factors occurs, a son or daughter may be motivated to urge that the parent move in with his or her family. This is not always the wisest course. For one thing, it frequently doesn't make either generation happy to live together; each has a different pace of life, and the older person may feel just as uncomfortable as the children and grandchildren. His or her chance of happiness may be improved if he or she has a place in the right residential-care facility—and has the opportunity to see the family as frequently as previously.

There is such a wide variety of residential-care facilities that it is impossible to present a guide for their selection here. One of the best resources for counseling and information is the Office of the Aging of the federal government, or of your state government. For counseling about local facilities, consult your family physician.

4. Foster homes.

In some communities, foster home-care programs have been set up to provide a family atmosphere for elderly persons who cannot live alone. These are particularly advantageous for the elderly person who needs some care and prefers a family atmosphere rather than an institutional setting. The patient in a foster home can take advantage of any home health services available in the community, just as if he were living in his own home. Check your local social-service agency to find out whether foster homes for the aging exist in your area.

5. Home health care.

Home health services bring to the patient's home medical, dental, nursing, social, and nutritional services, and physical, occupational, and speech therapy. An organized home-care program may be provided through a hospital, a visiting-nurse association, a public health department, or a for-profit agency (such as Upjohn Homemakers, Medical Personnel Pool, or Kelly Home Care Services). It should be ordered and directed by a physician and oriented specifically toward the individual patient's needs. It may reach the level of care provided in a skilled nursing home or it may simply combine the services of a homemaker with rehabilitative services in a nearby center.

Which persons are candidates for home health care? As a general rule, any person who is not acutely ill can be adequately tended in the home—provided his community agency offers a full range of home health services. If the person lives alone and requires constant care or supervision, he may be better off in a nursing home or in a residential-care facility—at lower cost than round-the-clock home coverage. If he lives alone but needs only intermittent care, he can obtain services ranging from "meals on wheels" to follow-up nursing care for a foot amputation. If the person lives with relatives who are willing to assist in his care, he can be managed at home even with such conditions as heart disease, cancer, diabetes, and mental illness.

As a rule of thumb the average family can manage an elderly disabled patient when:

(a)   He can move from bed to chair without being lifted.

(b)   He has normal or near-normal control of excretory functions.

(c)   He can take care of the essential elements of personal needs—eating, bathing, dressing, etc.

(d)   His mental condition is reasonably clear.

(e)   The medical-care program he needs can be adapted to the home.

Interestingly, at the same time that more and more institutions for long-term care of the aging are springing up, there is a trend toward development of organized home health services. Among the major reasons for this trend are: Home care makes it possible to release scarce hospital and nursing-home beds. Home-care costs (excluding round-the-clock service) are estimated to be considerably lower than inpatient-care costs. Home care provides a psychological benefit to many patients, compared to institutional care. Your physician can help you determine whether the person's home setting is physically and emotionally adapted to adequate care. He will also know which resources are available in a community.

6. *Day-care centers.*

More than two hundred centers for the chronically ill are now operating around the country, in this newest type of long-term-care service. Most day-care centers serve two types of patients: the severely disabled person who needs strong rehabilitative services, and the less severely disabled person who needs social and recreational orientation—a chance to be with other people instead of being a "shut-in."

Patients in day-care centers typically are there from nine to five, from two to five days a week. This type of care is also of a much lower level than that of a nursing home, but is appropriate to the situation. Costs run substantially below those of keeping a person in a nursing home.

Frequently, the decision about which type of long-term care should be used is not clear-cut. How do you decide about those chronically ill people who need some skilled nursing care, but who might be just as well off at home or in a residential-care facility? A starting principle is to *use personal resources first,* then institutional resources when personal resources are inadequate or unavailable. Second, the health goal for the person must be considered. If an effort is being made to *improve* his or her condition physically and mentally, then the patient is likely to require the kind of skilled care available at a nursing-care facility or through a home health program. A residential-care facility usually operates to maintain the status quo rather than to improve the patient's condition. Third, is the person too disabled to be adequately nursed at home by relatives and/or a home health service? Or, are the people at home capable of ministering to the patient's needs? Fourth, is the presence of a patient requiring constant care a disruptive factor in the home? Fifth, does the patient recognize that a nursing home will enable him or her to heighten comfort and/or ability to function?

Suppose an elderly person isn't capable of making the final decision on a move by himself or herself—how can you help? Don't ask whether or not he or she wants to make a move. If the person says "no," you may be in the difficult position of having to overrule the decision. Enlist the help of the family doctor or a social worker to help explain the need for a move. Make the decision firmly, using the support of the doctor, and move quickly toward a "trial" stay in the facility. The "trial" will, in most instances, turn out to be a permanent stay, with the willing agreement (or insistence) of the patient.

CHAPTER

22

WHAT TO LOOK FOR
IN A NURSING HOME

ANNABELLE JASPER IS SEVENTY-EIGHT YEARS OLD. SHE HAS
been at Marcy Hills Nursing Home for just over four years.
She had been living with her married daughter, Beatrice,
when she fell and broke her hip. Beatrice had decided she
just couldn't manage an invalid woman and four children
at the same time. And Beatrice's husband never was very
keen about having his mother-in-law, who had a rather
sharp tongue, under the same roof with him. All things
considered, Annabelle Jasper is doing fairly well at Marcy
Hills. True, she seldom gets out of her wheelchair any more,
her memory is going, and she is confused some of the time.
But the nurses have standing orders to give her tranquilizers
whenever necessary, she seems to get good food, and the
staff seems to be very kind. The doctor drops in once every
month or two, and Annabelle's daughter comes in about as
often; it's been six months since she saw any of the grandchildren. But she seems to enjoy chatting with her room-
mate and she watches television a great deal.

Annabelle Jasper could be a composite of hundreds of
thousands of nursing-home patients across the country, and
Marcy Hills might be typical of many of those nursing
homes . . . not good, not bad. If you have an Annabelle

Jasper in your family, and have decided that a nursing home is the best place for her, how do you decide which nursing home?

There has been a tremendous increase in the number and types of nursing homes in recent years. Franchised organizations have opened brand new motel-type facilities in many communities. Physicians and enterpreneurs have been opening nursing homes to serve the needs of the sick and aging. Nonprofit charitable or religious organizations continue to operate facilities, as do independent nursing-home owners.

Services and costs range widely, making the choice more difficult. In this chapter and in the accompanying checklist you will find guidelines in six major areas: the patient's needs, services offered, physical plant, livability, licensing and accreditation, and costs.

1. *The patient's needs.* Unfortunately, the patient's needs don't always get put at the top of the list, because the need to put someone in a nursing home is often precipitated by a crisis. It may be that an elderly person is hospitalized and only toward discharge time does the family recognize that the aged parent cannot be taken care of at home. Or the care-taker-relative suddenly gets sick. Or the elderly person, who has been living alone, leaves the stove on by accident, or becomes paranoid, provoking an emergency call from the landlord to the children. It is important to remember that, even in a crisis, the aged parent still deserves consideration as a person and a chance to voice his or her own views.

A family conference may be in order, with the patient and his or her physician present. The focus should be on which nursing-care facility might be best for her needs, rather than on whether or not to use such a facility. The advice of a social worker can be very helpful at this point.

Your first concern should be to identify the patient's specific needs. Does she have a physical disability or multiple chronic illnesses? How much nursing care does she require? Is she depressed and unhappy? Will she need a special diet, physical therapy, psychiatric care? An elderly person entering a nursing home has the right to feel that there is still a chance to live a happy and useful, though limited, life. She needs reassurance of her own worth and the fact that other people care. Another important point to consider is the older person's ethnic or religious background. She has good reason to feel insecure about this move to a strange place late in life. It will help if she finds herself among other elderly people with a similar background.

2. *Services offered.* The level of medical, nursing, rehabilitative, and social services in a nursing home varies widely. Here are basic elements to look for:

a. Every home should have a medical director who helps set policies and arrange for emergency calls. Each attending physician should plan to see the patient at the request of the patient, the family, or nursing home personnel, or whenever the patient's condition indicates—in any case, at least monthly.

b. Every home should have a nursing staff that understands basic techniques used to prevent deformity and muscle contracture, to retrain the patient in self-care, to assist the incontinent patient in regaining bowel and bladder control. In a skilled nursing home of seventy-five beds or more, an R.N. should be in duty at all times; in a smaller home, an L.P.N. (Licensed Practical Nurse) or L.V.N. (Licensed Vocational Nurse) may substitute part of the time.

c. Every home should have a full- or part-time licensed physical therapist in charge of a prescribed physical-therapy and rehabilitation program; a trained dietitian; and access to psychiatric counseling.

d. Every home should have a social and recreational program that encourages patients to develop relationships with others, managed by trained social-service personnel.

e. Every home should have sufficient personnel to give active, not just passive, care to patients. Most good skilled-nursing-care facilities have roughly one employee for every two patients. The treatment received by incontinent patients is one clue to adequate staffing in relation to the quality of care. Ask (through your doctor if necessary) whether most patients are trained or retrained to normal bladder function rather than using a catheter; the latter is a low-cost convenience for the nursing home on a long-term basis. The best facilities really work hard at the little things: for example, a rehabilitation program that concentrates on simple, basic activities that we all take for granted, seemingly as trivial as moving from a wheelchair to a toilet and back, or walking a few steps to a dining table. These independent functions make a world of difference to the patient.

3. *Physical plant.* A well-planned, attractive building is essential to good care in a nursing home; but don't give undue importance to brightly colored carpets, drapes, and walls. Bricks, mortar, and decor are less important than good professional services and special features for the safety and convenience of the elderly patient.

Look for these elements in the building's design:

a. A minimum of 80 square feet per patient bed, with no more than four beds in a room

b. 100 square feet minimum for a private room

c. Another 50 square feet of space per bed for recreation and dining, for 75 percent of the beds in the home

d. Bathrooms or lavatories adjoining bedrooms if possible

e. Lighting adequate for elderly persons with impaired vision

f. Handrails in halls and stairwells

g. Effective call systems, with outlets for each bed

h. Beds equipped with rails

i. Bathrooms equipped with grab rails and a call buzzer

j. Benches or chairs in hallways

k. Travel distances of not more than 100–150 feet from any room to the dayroom, dining room, or elevator

l. At least two easily accessible independent exits on each wing or floor

m. Unobstructed corridors at least seven feet wide

n. A sprinkler system or other fire-protection system and an alarm-and-evacuation plan that is tested periodically

o. A well-kept and protected area for walking or sitting outside of the building

4. *Livability.* The purpose of the nursing home is to improve the old person's quality of living. Watch out for this: If the home is spotless, odorless, has little patient movement and no signs of discontent—that is a place where the inmates are just waiting to die. When there are sounds, kitchen or cooking smells, and small-group activity—those old people are taking some pleasure from their lives.

Look for a "homey" atmosphere. Grandmother is not likely to feel very comfortable in an impersonal institution.

Rooms and halls should be clean and *relatively* free of odor (*not* antiseptic!). The patients should be neatly dressed and communicating with each other and with members of the staff. The lounge should have a warm feeling about it— you can sense that by the way the patients use it. In particular, look for the presence of volunteers, and for cheerful responses to the patients by volunteers and staff members. Requests to them by the patients should be answered without undue delay. (Too often, a patient is left sitting too long in a wheelchair or on a commode, because the staff is "too busy.")

Food preparation and mealtimes are important to check out. A quick inspection of the kitchen can indicate if the food is being prepared under hygienic conditions. Food texture and color are important, since elderly patients often have poor appetites; wholesome or not, food that is unappealing may prompt them to stop eating entirely. Meeting for meals is *the* major social activity for many nursing-home residents, and being able to get together in a pleasant dining room is a significant daily experience.

To determine whether the home has made a successful effort to avoid a dehumanized, institutional aura, see if you can answer the following questions affirmatively:

Are people permitted or even encouraged to have a favorite chair or other furniture in their rooms?

Is visiting permitted throughout the day and evening?

Is there an area for visiting in private, if a person does not have a private room?

Is the place decorated like a home, with familiar colors and materials, rather than like an institution?

Are there recreational or even occupational opportunities for nearly every resident? Even an irreversibly senile patient confined to a wheelchair can take pleasure in doing something she has always done—knitting, for instance. In some nursing homes, patients even find themselves employed (at low wages) for doing contractual work for private business firms, such as sorting and packing of merchandise.

Finally, look for little things that help patients preserve their sense of dignity. Some nursing homes provide special implements, such as a plate with a metal rim against which food can be pushed; forks and spoons with oversized handles; suction pads to keep a plate fixed on the table; a long-handled comb and brush.

5. *Licensing and accreditation.* Most nursing homes are privately owned. More than half the nursing-home beds in this country are in buildings that have been constructed within the last ten years. These two factors alone make it difficult to follow any uniform set of standards, and make it imperative that you conduct your own personal inspection of a home. Look for evidence of some form of licensing and/or accreditation; but don't be 100 percent guided by it. State and local licensing laws vary widely and may not insure that a home meets modern standards of care.

Better than most state or local licensing is accreditation

under a program conducted by the Joint Commission on Accreditation of Hospitals, where a nursing home must submit to periodic inspections covering medical and nursing services and physical plant. Medicare provides another measure of a nursing home. Only homes that meet certain minimal standards are approved for Medicare patients—but enforcement of the standards has not been uniformly maintained. Finally, affiliation with one or more accredited hospitals may give evidence that the home is providing reasonably adequate care.

Ask the nursing-home administrator for evidence of participation in any of these programs—but don't be overly impressed by the presence or absence of such evidence. Most well-run nursing homes are licensed, but many are not approved by Medicare or by the Joint Commission on Accreditation of Hospitals.

6. *Costs.* The price of nursing-home care will be a major consideration for most families. Good care is not cheap, but it may be cheaper in the long run than low-cost, poor-quality care.

Staffing is the costliest item in a nursing home. Inadequately staffed homes may allow an elderly person to lie in bed for days because it is easier than getting him up, dressed, and exercised. The result can be physical and mental deterioration that requires more expensive hospitalization, drug therapy, and special intensive-care services. Add to this the anguish of seeing a human being go downhill instead of maintaining maximum independence and self-help. The perspective on cost should be relative to the care that is given.

Your next step is to analyze the available sources of finances. Is the patient eligible for Medicare coverage? What other health insurance does the patient have? (See Chapters 23 and 24.) Will Medicaid or other state or local aid programs pay part or all of the bill? Your local welfare agency can help you answer this last question. Add whatever resources the elderly person may have, or whatever you and/or other family members can contribute per month, and you have a basic figure to work with.

Remember that the nursing home's basic rate will cover only room, board, and routine nursing service. You must add any extras such as charges for private accommodations, linen, personal laundry, hair care, foot care, dental care, glasses, hearing aids, special nursing, special diets, drugs, etc. You should be able to get a reasonable estimate from the home of what these costs might be for the specific patient —at least for the short term.

Projections into the future also should be included in your cost estimates. Is it likely that the patient will require nursing-home care for the balance of his or her life? If so, should a longtime family home and/or furnishings be sold? Or is there a chance that he or she will recover sufficiently to be moved to a less expensive residential facility, or back home with the support of a home-care program? You will need the help of a doctor in making this forecast, and in revising it periodically.

After reviewing these guidelines, develop a list of nursing homes that might be suitable for the patient. The doctor and community social-service agencies are your major sources of information; the doctor can identify homes which he or his colleagues routinely visit, and which he feels come closest to meeting the patient's needs. Remember that if you choose a home that the patient's physician does not routinely visit, it may be necessary to select another physician to provide continuing care. The social-service agencies may be better equipped than the doctor to help with questions of cost and livability.

You may want to cross-check their suggestions with a minister, a visiting nurse, or another health professional, such as a physical therapist who regularly visits nursing homes in your area. Next, before a crisis arises, visit at least two or three of the homes yourself, armed with the questions raised in this chapter and in the accompanying checklist. Use the checklist to give you some comparative rating of the homes you visit. Note the pluses; but also check for minuses indicated in the trouble-signs sections of the checklist.

Plan your visit so you can be there when a meal is served. Try to chat with some of the nursing staff and the patients as well as with the administrator. Don't be afraid to ask questions. At stake are the health and happiness of your relative for a good many months or even years to come.

NURSING-HOME CHECKLIST

(Indicate *Yes* or *No*)

Services	Home #1	Home #2	Home #3
Medical director			
Physician available in emergencies			
Emergency transportation available			
Dental care available			
Physical therapy available			
Occupational and speech therapy available			
Program to prevent muscle contracture			
Self-care training program			
Special diets			
Medications as prescribed			
X-ray and lab services available			
Social and recreational program			
Services available meet needs			
Hospital affiliation			
Staff			
Nursing service around the clock			
Registered nurses available			
Patient charts available and up to date			

Services	(Indicate *Yes* or *No*) Home #1	Home #2	Home #3
Nurse call by each bed			
Staff members respond quickly and cheerfully to patient calls			
Staff neatly dressed, courteous			
Patients friendly with staff			
Food			
Kitchen clean, well organized			
Menus varied			
Menus appealing, well balanced			
Portions adequate			
Meals carefully served			
Building			
Fire resistant and/or sprinkler system			
Frequent fire drills			
Exits well marked			
Building in good repair			
Well lighted			
Homey atmosphere			
Rooms and halls clean, cheery			
Rooms not cramped			
Fresh sheets on bed			
Easily accessible bath, toilet			
Comfortable lounge			
Recreation rooms			
Facilities for special therapy			
Relatively free of odor			
Livability			
Patients are clean, neatly dressed			
Patients look alive, interested			

Services	(Indicate *Yes* or *No*)		
	Home #1	Home #2	Home #3
Good interchange between patients, staff			
Patients eat together and communicate			
Patients use lounge, recreation areas			
Facilities for visits from friends, relatives			
Barber, hairdresser available			
Help for patients in shopping, correspondence			
Religious contacts available			
Favorite furniture allowed			
Licensing/accreditation			
Licensing or accreditation certificates posted			
Joint Commission on Accreditation of Hospitals			
Medicare-approved			
State-licensed			
Locally-licensed			

CHAPTER

23

WHAT YOU NEED TO KNOW ABOUT HEALTH INSURANCE

JOE BERNSTEIN, HENRY HEIDE, AND MARGARET BRUCATTI shared one problem in common: all had incurred spinal injuries and had had a competent neurosurgeon remove a crushed disc. All were about the same age, in their early forties, all spent about three weeks in the hospital, on two different occasions, and all recovered satisfactorily from their operations. But when it came to paying the bill, the similarities ended.

Joe's care was completely covered; he belonged to a health maintenance organization (HMO), which paid for everything except the magazines Joe purchased from the hospital "drugstore" cart.

Henry, who ran his own one-man accounting firm, didn't fare so well; his major-medical policy covered about 75 percent of his bills, but Henry still was obligated to pay the doctor and the hospital a total of $2,500.

Margaret, a secretary with a large corporation, was responsible personally for a total of $600: $100 of the hospital bill, $400 of the surgeon's bill, and $100 worth of prescription drugs. Insurance covered the remaining $9,000.

Even though seven out of ten Americans currently have some form of private health insurance, the benefits and coverages vary tremendously. As the costs of medical care rise more rapidly than the cost of living, most families are increasingly concerned to make sure that their health insurance is adequate to protect them against unexpected expense. Health insurance traditionally has covered most hospital bills and surgical procedures to some extent. In recent years, more and more people have added coverage for major-medical benefits in the hospital and to a lesser extent in physicians' offices. Only recently has there been a government-supported drive to promote almost complete comprehensive coverage for all medical bills, including preventive care, through health maintenance organizations.

The purpose of health insurance is to pool the risk of illness among a number of people. It pays for services that are needed some of the time by some of the people, while the cost is borne by all the people who pay for insurance.

In this chapter and the next, on the government's Medicaid and Medicare programs, you will find brief explanations and guidelines to help you understand, select, and make the most of the health-insurance coverages available. Frequently the decision as to the type and extent of health coverage is made by an employer or union. Even if you find yourself in this situation, you should be fully informed about the coverage you and your family have, and should investigate the possibility of optional or supplemental coverage if you feel that is desirable.

How much coverage should you have? One hundred percent? Ninety-five percent? Eighty percent? Fifty percent? Time was when most people were satisfied to have their hospital and surgical bills covered, because other costs of medical care didn't seem big enough to need insurance. Then, in the 1960's and early 1970's, as health-care costs escalated rapidly, health-insurance coverage broadened. Policies were readily available to pay "first dollar" costs, meaning that from the time you walked into a doctor's office until you were discharged from the hospital, your medical and surgical bills were covered. Additional coverage has been added for prescription drugs, for eyeglasses, for hearing aids, for psychiatric care, for dental care, and for preventive care. But as the coverage increased, so did the cost of health insurance. Now it's time to challenge whether such complete coverage is really the "best buy" for individuals or for the American public.

In general, "first dollar" coverage is costly and tends to encourage unnecessary use of medical-care services by both patients and physicians. The *"best buy,"* in my view, is a policy under which the insured family pays the first $50–$200 of medical-care costs out of pocket, and picks up a 20-percent share of the next $2,000–$5,000 of costs with the insurance paying 80 percent. The family pays nothing over the $2,000–$5,000 limit, with all additional medical-care costs covered by insurance, to a maximum of $1 million over a lifetime. The extent of coverage should be broad, including visits to physicians' offices, hospital and nursing-home care, home health care, psychiatric care, and preventive care. Too many health-insurance policies today discriminate against the lower-cost care that can be rendered in a physician's office. The worst example is the exclusion of outpatient psychiatric care in many policies, which cover such care only in an expensive hospital setting.

This recommended package is likely to be lower in premium costs than first-dollar coverage. (If not, beware restrictions on the benefits.) It encourages patients to be careful in their initial decisions to seek medical care, but at the same time insures that if there is a medical catastrophe, the family will not be paying more than $500–$1,500 of the costs of care.

Before an emergency strikes, analyze your health-insurance coverage by getting out your policies, reading and understanding the benefits listed, and paying particular attention to the *exclusions* set forth in the policies. Usually these tell you more than the benefits do! And don't be influenced by a high or low premium alone; the total package is important. Following is a list of major points to look for in your own coverage. If these are not present, talk to your employer, your union, or your insurance agent about adding any missing items. (You *can* influence your coverage by speaking up.)

1. *Hospitalization coverage.* This should include complete payment for room and board for semiprivate accommodations, plus complete payment for use of such hospital facilities as the operating room, X rays, laboratory, intensive-care units, and special services in orthopedics and shock therapy. You should not expect your insurance to cover "hotel extras" such as telephone service, nor will the hospital coverage take care of the physicians' fees for interpretation of X rays and lab tests.

2. *Surgical expenses.* These should be completely covered for both office and hospital surgery, except plastic surgery for cosmetic purposes.

3. *Maternity benefits.* Coverage for prenatal and postnatal services, plus delivery, should be routine in any policy. If you have a teenage daughter, check to determine whether the policy would cover her if she became pregnant while still a dependent.

4. *Diagnostic tests.* More and more policies now are including coverage for laboratory tests, X rays, electrocardiograms, and other diagnostic procedures, whether performed in or out of the hospital. A good policy should offer such benefits as a means of keeping patients *out* of the hospital.

5. *Home and office visits.* You should have coverage to protect against high frequency of visits for chronic illness or for a lengthy, acute illness. Outpatient visits to rehabilitation centers, for physical or occupational therapy, are often covered under this provision.

6. *Medications.* Most policies today cover drugs given in the hospital; a few cover prescriptions written in the doctor's office. The latter type of coverage can be a protection against costly drug bills related to a chronic condition. Coverage for blood transfusions may be unnecessary if your community has a good blood-bank program.

7. *Psychiatric care.* Look for a policy that will cover office visits to a psychiatrist as well as treatment in a psychiatric hospital. (Warning: Some policies pay for office visits, but limit the payments to 10–20 percent of the charges.)

8. *Orthopedic braces, crutches, and prosthetic appliances.* You should have coverage for any of these when prescribed by a physician. Coverage for eyeglasses, contact lenses, and hearing aids is increasing.

9. *Nursing care.* Most policies cover skilled nursing care, but not custodial care, in a nursing home. Many others cover private-duty nurses at home or in the hospital as long as R.N.'s are employed. Unfortunately, few policies cover the services of less expensive nursing personnel such as practical nurses or home health aides. This type of coverage is worth having. It can save more expensive institutional care. Almost no policies cover housekeeping or meal-preparation services at home, unfortunately.

10. *Dental care.* This seems to be the fastest growing new form of insurance, sometimes included in broad-coverage medical/hospital plans and sometimes sold separately. Policies are available for routine care only or may be expanded to include root-canal work, orthodontic care, and replacement of dentures. Routine care includes X rays, oral exams, cleaning, treatment of dental defects or diseases, and fillings.

The next step in evaluating your health-insurance program is to determine whether or not your policy will pay for most of the costs incurred, or only a small percentage of them. Simply having coverage for a specific service does not always mean that a health-insurance company will pay the whole bill. There are two basic factors affecting how much your health insurance will pay for: length of coverage and type of coverage.

Length of coverage. Check your policies to determine how long a time period is provided for each benefit covered. For example, your coverage for hospitalization should be, if possible, for 365 days or longer. A policy that limits hospital benefits to 30 or 60 days can deprive you of coverage for a catastrophic illness just when you need it most. Coverage for physicians' visits should not be limited to one per month or five per span of illness. Those are the kinds of restrictions you find in low-cost, highly promoted policies.

Type of coverage. Health-insurance plans generally offer one or more of three types of coverage: service benefits, indemnity benefits, or major-medical benefits. Here is what these terms mean.

1. *Service benefits.* This type of coverage provides for full payment of covered services rendered by participating providers. For example, a Blue Cross policy usually pays the full cost of hospital room and board in a semiprivate room, regardless of whether the hospital charges $175 or $350 a day. Blue Shield policies generally provide service benefits for physicians' services, although sometimes only when the subscriber and/or family earnings are less than the annual income specified in the policy.

In certain policies, a Blue Shield allowance may represent full payment for an appendectomy as long as your income is under $8,000 a year. In this situation, the surgeon has agreed with Blue Shield to accept its standard allowance, say $275, for income levels below $8,000. If your income were over $8,000, however, and if the surgeon's fee were higher than the standard payment allowed by Blue Shield, you would be responsible for paying the difference. This is also the case if the surgeon is a nonparticipating physician; a nonparticipating physician is not obligated to accept Blue Shield's payment allowance. If you have a Blue Shield policy providing full service benefits, check with your physician to determine whether he is a participating physician or not.

If you do not have full service benefits, make sure that you have a major-medical policy (see below) to cover excess charges.

2. *Indemnity benefits.* This term describes specific cash payments for each benefit provided. For example, an indem-

nity policy may provide payment of $50 a day for hospital room and board, $100 for the surgical fee for an appendectomy, or $10 for a consultation with a medical specialist— no matter what the usual charge for these services may be.

On the surface this looks like a bad program. It appears as if the patient will hold the bag for any medical-care costs exceeding a generally low payment schedule. However, an indemnity plan does offer one specific advantage: a guaranteed premium. Because the health-insurance company can predict its costs fairly accurately, and does not have to speculate on possible increases in hospital rates and doctors' fees, it can afford to offer coverage at a reasonably low cost without the possibility of a rate increase. The indemnity benefit examples I have used are very low. Some indemnity policies do have schedules that pay almost the prevailing rate, while others pay so little as to be virtually useless. The buyer should find out what the daily hospital rates are in his area before purchasing such coverage.

Caution: An indemnity plan may provide a low-cost base for your health-insurance coverage; but it should always be coupled with a major-medical plan to insure you against financial disaster. For example, the total cost of a relatively simple operation for removal of varicose veins might be about $2,000 for hospital and surgical services. An indemnity plan might pay as little as $500, leaving the patient to pay the balance.

3. *Major-medical benefits.* A major-medical policy might be compared to an umbrella. It will keep most of the rain off your head, even though your feet may get slightly wet. It does this by paying a high percentage of the costs covered, but not 100 percent of them.

You can buy a major-medical policy by itself, or you can buy it to supplement a limited-service benefit plan or an indemnity plan. As a rule, most major-medical policies require you to pay out of your own pocket a certain amount, called the "deductible," which usually ranges from $100– $500 in any calendar year. After that, the policy will pay 75–

80 percent of all costs related to covered benefits, to a maximum.

The policy will not reimburse you for benefits already paid by a limited service or indemnity plan. Looking again at the example of the varicose-vein operation mentioned above, let's assume that the indemnity plan paid $500—leaving a balance of $1,500. The major-medical plan might require that you pay the next $100. Of the remaining $1,400, the major-medical plan would pay 80 percent, or $1,120; you would pay the other $280. Of the total $2,000 bill, you would pay $380, and your two insurance plans would pay the balance.

Caution: Major-medical plans have limitations to watch for. Most impose a maximum benefit per lifetime. Today this limit should be at least $250,000, and preferably $1,000,000, to make sure that a serious, long-term illness will be well covered. Don't rely on a plan with a $50,000 maximum. One major illness or accident could use that up in a year. However, sometimes you can get an excess-coverage liability policy—one that picks up after $25,000 or $50,000—for a relatively low extra premium.

Additional cautions regarding limitations of policies:

Check to see whether the deductibles and the maximum benefits are specified per individual or per family. Deductibles per family cost you more; maximum benefits per individual protect you better.

Check to see whether the deductible is on a per-illness or per-year basis. The latter is preferable.

Note whether a "preexisting" condition—that is, an illness that existed before insurance coverage took effect—will ever be covered or whether you must always be responsible for payment of these bills *in toto.* Some policies pick up coverage after six months to one year.

Determine whether your dependents covered under the policy include children from birth through age twenty-five. If not, make sure that some coverage is obtained when the policy no longer includes them.

Determine whether the policy pays the doctor or hospital directly (usually so in the case of Blue Shield and Blue Cross) or pays you. In the latter case, you have the responsibility for paying the physician and the hospital, and collecting from the insurance carrier. (If the carrier feels the physician's fee is too high, it may reduce it or not pay at all.) You should press the physician and the hospital to sign the claim form quickly so as to speed the reimbursement process, and make sure the bill appears reasonable.

Check to make sure your health insurance covers work-related illness and injury if you do not have workman's compensation insurance.

The newest widely available coverage, technically considered a prepayment plan rather than an insurance plan, comes through joining a health maintenance organization. Through participating physicians and hospitals, an HMO offers a broad range of basic health services for a fixed monthly premium. These usually include: physicians' services, hospital services, emergency health services, short-term outpatient mental health services, diagnostic services, home health services and preventive health services. In general, HMOs offer a broader range of benefits than traditional Blue Cross-Blue Shield or private insurance policies. The federal government has financed the development of a number of HMOs around the country, the best-known of which are organized around group practices such as Kaiser Permanente in California, Group Health Cooperative of Puget Sound (Seattle) and Health Insurance Plan of Greater New York (HIP). In some cases, groups of physicians practicing separately have agreed to participate in an HMO serving their community. These physicians may continue with traditional practices for other patients, who are covered by private health insurance, while at the same time providing a comprehensive range of services to HMO members.

If an HMO has received federal approval, large employers in that community are required to offer employees the option of choosing health-care coverage under the HMO or under a traditional insurance plan, so long as the costs to the company are the same. In most cases, however, the premiums for participation in an HMO are higher than standard insurance coverage, since the HMO offers a more comprehensive package with fewer exclusions. Employees may pay the difference, or individuals or families may enroll separately.

The advantages of an HMO are: Comprehensive coverage, including preventive care, is available for all family members. Participating doctors tend to seek to manage the costs of care more efficiently, since their HMO income is probably dependent not only on the number of services they render but on how well they manage to reduce high-cost care, such as hospitalization and surgery. An HMO may be the best bet for an individual or family who cannot get group insurance coverage through an employer or union or trade association. (Individual health-insurance policies, either through Blue Cross-Blue Shield or through private companies, tend to be very costly and have somewhat limited benefits in comparison.)

On the negative side, HMO premiums tend to cost more than other policies. Your choice of physicians or hospitals is also restricted to those who have agreed to participate. Finally, in some large group-practice HMOs, care tends to become impersonal.

Once you've evaluated your policies and your needs, how can you improve your coverage if necessary? Most people have their basic health-insurance coverage through a group plan with an employer or a union. Find out who in your company or union handles the insurance plan and ask whether any improvement in the coverage is planned. Ask if it's possible to obtain extended benefits under the same group plan by paying the additional premium yourself; some policies permit employees to purchase additional coverage if they wish. Ask if an HMO is coming into existence in the area.

If you don't have health insurance through a company

or union plan, or if these plans are inadequate, consider extending your coverage in other ways:

1. If you belong to trade or fraternal organizations, they often have group health-insurance plans costing less than an individual policy. Insurance companies write more benefits into group plans, too.

2. Call your local Blue Cross-Blue Shield representatives. These are nonprofit, prepayment plans operated with the support of hospitals and physicians across the country. Blue Cross and Blue Shield often give nongroup subscribers more extensive coverage, including service benefits, than are available from commercial health insurance companies. In most areas, Blue Cross and Blue Shield also offer major-medical benefits.

3. Call your local insurance agent. After you have information about the health insurance available from organizations to which you belong, or from Blue Cross and Blue Shield, ask the agent to recommend a policy that will offer the coverage suggested earlier in this chapter.

4. Mail-order insurance. Through newspaper ads and direct mail, many insurance companies offer various plans for individuals. Some offer special protection against one dreaded disease only, such as cancer. These, though inexpensive, are probably not worth the investment, which would be better applied to broader health-insurance coverage. Other mail-order plans may give you an adequate base of indemnity insurance at reasonable cost, but be wary. Before committing yourself to a purchase, send for a copy of the policy and compare the benefits with those of Blue Cross and Blue Shield. If the program looks good, check on the standing of the mail-order company with your local Better Business Bureau, your state insurance commissioner (if you buy from a carrier in your own state, you generally have more protection), or the Health Insurance Association of America (750 Third Avenue, New York City).

If you must buy coverage as an individual to match the

benefits recommended here, the cost may well be more than your family budget can stand. That's why it's so important to utilize group policies whenever they are available. Individuals usually must pay premiums on a community-rated basis, which means that the costs are averaged across the region in which you live. Most group policies are purchased on an experience-rated basis, which means that premiums are based on the actual health-care costs of the insured group only. Since most insured groups are made up of younger, healthy workers and their families, the costs—and premiums—tend to be lower than those of the community at large, which includes older people and less healthy people.

A few pointers on buying individual policies, if you have no group available to you: Make sure your policy is noncancelable, even if it costs you a bit more. Otherwise you could be out in the cold just when you need protection the most. If you are leaving a group policy, check to see whether you are guaranteed conversion to an individual health-insurance policy. The benefits may be less, but there should be no waiting period for coverage. Look for a policy that doesn't exclude preexisting disease permanently. Most individual policies do permit an exclusion to be lifted on application from the insured person. (Exclusions usually apply to diseases of an organ—say the kidney—rather than simply to a disease itself—such as kidney stones.)

If coverage must be cut down because of cost factors, your best bet is to buy a major-medical policy against catastrophic illness. It might have a $500 deductible each year, and then pay 75 percent of all hospital, surgical, and medical expenses over that amount up to a lifetime maximum of $250,000.

And if cost is no object, don't overinsure. For the most part, insurance carriers coordinate benefits and payments with each other. One policy will be the lead policy, paying first; other policies can then pick up any deductibles or leftovers—but rarely will benefits exceed the actual expenses incurred.

GUIDELINES FOR FAMILY COVERAGE

The American Academy of Pediatrics has developed the following guidelines to help you select a good insurance program for your family from the great variety of policies available, or to aid you in improving your present policy.

A. *Features That Are Essential to Any Sound Health-Insurance Policy:*

1. All members of a family should be covered equally, including each child from birth.
2. Provision should be made to cover all major-medical and surgical expenses.
3. Provision should be made for protection from catastrophic health expenses.
4. Provision should be made for converting and continuing a health-insurance policy when the subscriber terminates his employment.
5. Exclusions should be clearly identified and completely understood.
6. The health-insurance policy or the insurance agent should explain the meaning of coinsurance, corridors, or deductibles if they are a facet of your policy. The total out-of-pocket expenditure that the policy owner could incur should be clearly stated.

B. *Priorities:*

Comprehensive health-insurance coverage will change with changes in medical technology, but the following are benefits that should be covered in a comprehensive medical-insurance policy.

1. First Priorities:
   a. Medical care to include health supervision and preventive care supervised by a physician, wherever performed.
   b. Surgical care, wherever performed, and the diag-

nosis of injury, illness, or disease. Plastic or reconstructive surgery where necessary to restore
function or the emotional well-being of an individual.

  c. Pregnancy should be wholly or partially included.
All complications of pregnancy must be covered,
including the care of the unborn child.

  d. Care of the newborn infant from *birth*. (Many
policies exclude infants for two weeks to thirty
days.)

  e. Laboratory and pathological services requested by
a physician and performed in an approved laboratory.

  f. X-ray services wherever performed.

  g. Radiation therapy wherever performed.

  h. Anesthesia services.

  i. Consultations wherever performed.

  j. Concurrent care (services rendered to a patient by
more than one physician).

  k. Inhalation and physical therapy under the direction of a physician.

  l. Drugs while in a hospital, and other drug costs
beyond an annual deductible.

  m. Emergency psychiatric care.

  n. Emergency ambulance service.

  o. Extended-care services ordered by a physician.

  p. Prosthetic appliances, braces.

2. Second Priorities:

  a. Psychiatric services.

  b. Podiatry.

  c. Rental or purchase of medical equipment.

  d. Psychological testing.

3. Third Priorities:

  a. Cosmetic surgery (elective).

  b. Transplantations (nonexperimental).

  c. Eyeglasses.

  d. Social services, if beneficial, and overall medical
care of the patient.

24

TIPS ON MEDICARE AND MEDICAID COVERAGE

MORE THAN 40 MILLION AMERICANS HAVE SOME OR ALL OF their care paid for by the two major government health-care financing programs, Medicare and Medicaid. Because these programs primarily cover the elderly and the poor, levels of confusion over what is paid for—and what isn't—are higher than with any other form of health insurance or prepayment plan. For example:

Henry Visinsky, a seventy-five-year-old retired plumber, was very upset when his family doctor told him that his shortness of breath was due to emphysema, a chronic, irre-versible lung condition. The doctor advised Henry to stop smoking and to start some simple exercises to maintain what breathing capacity he had left. Henry didn't want to accept the verdict; he asked for another opinion. His doctor sent him to a nearby lung specialist, who confirmed the diag-nosis and encouraged Henry to accept his disease and learn to live with it. Henry was even more upset when he re-ceived a bill for seventy-five dollars from the pulmonary specialist, submitted it to Medicare, and was refused re-imbursement for 80 percent of his payment. Medicare officials told him that the second opinion didn't qualify as a "con-sultation" under Medicare rules; a "consultation" has to be requested by the doctor, not by the patient, and must include a formal report back to the first doctor. Henry is still breathing hard over that bureaucratic interpretation.

Victoria Summers, eighty-six, had been living alone until she had a bad fall accompanied by an unexplained episode of gastrointestinal bleeding. She was hospitalized for three weeks and then was ready for discharge to a nursing home. When her daughter went to pay the hospital bill, she was informed that there was no bill to pay. Medicare was taking care of most of the bill, and Medicaid was paying the other $350 in charges that weren't covered by Medicare. The daughter, angry to have her mother considered "on welfare," struggled for three months to get the decision reversed so that she could pay the $350. The family was not wealthy, but certainly neither was it poor. Victoria's daughter rightly felt that there were many other more needy people who could use the benefits of Medicaid financing for their health care, so she didn't accept the windfall as many others might have. She later learned that her mother, when asked by a social worker to state her income, had replied "None of your business!" The social worker had chosen to write "none" on the hospital financial form under "annual income," and the billing office automatically filed a Medicaid request for payment.

Because Medicare and Medicaid are huge public programs, run by bureaucrats in federal and state governments, there is a complex maze of rules and regulations that leads to countless situations similar to those above—many of which are more damaging and more costly. If you or your relatives may be eligible for Medicare or Medicaid benefits, the following tips can save you some aggravation. (Just to get this information from appropriate agencies, we must have made at least half a dozen phone calls and talked to twenty different people!)

1. *Definitions.* Medicare is a federal health-insurance program for people sixty-five and over, consisting of hospital and medical coverage. Part A is compulsory hospitalization insurance, financed by contributions from employees and

employers under the Social Security system. Part B is supplementary medical insurance to pay for physicians' services
and some other medical services not covered by Part A; it
is financed by monthly premiums shared equally by those
who voluntarily sign up for the program and by the federal
government. The Medicare program is also extended to certain disabled people under sixty-five who have been entitled
to Social Security disability payments for at least two con-
secutive years, as well as those suffering from chronic renal
(kidney) disease.

The Medicaid program (Medical, in California) is a combined federal- and state-financed program to pay for health
care for persons whose income and resources are regarded as
insufficient, regardless of their age. This particularly includes
supplementary payments for persons over sixty-five; the blind,
the disabled, and members of families with dependent children. Some states include, at state expense, other needy and
low-income people. All of the money to pay for Medicaid
comes from federal, state, and local taxes.

2. *Benefits.* Medicare Part A, or hospital insurance,
provides basic protection against the costs of inpatient hospital care, up to certain limits, and for post-hospital skilled
nursing care and post-hospital home health care, again up to
certain limits. The hospital insurance pays for inpatient hospital bills, except for a deductible amount * payable by the
patient in each benefit period. Part B of Medicare pays 80
percent of medical and surgical "reasonable" charges after
the insured individual has paid a deductible * on these
charges. It provides supplemental protection against the costs
of physicians' services, medical services and supplies, home
health-care services, outpatient hospital services, therapy, and
certain other services.

Medicaid benefits vary from state to state (except Arizona,
which has no plan). These services, at least, are always included: inpatient hospital care, outpatient hospital services,
other laboratory and X-ray services, skilled-nursing-facility

* These deductibles change in amount every year or two.

services, physician services, screening, diagnosis, and treatment of children under twenty-one, home health-care services, and family-planning services. In many states Medicaid also pays for dental care, prescribed drugs, eyeglasses, clinic services, and other diagnostic, screening, preventive, and rehabilitative services. Medicaid can pay what Medicare does not, if people are eligible for both programs. For example, if Henry Visinsky were eligible for Medicaid as well as Medicare, the second opinion would probably have been paid for by Medicaid.

3. *Doctor's charges.* Neither Medicare nor Medicaid pay the usual and customary fee of most doctors. "Reasonable" reimbursement levels by the federal government are set at the lowest of the physician's actual charge, his customary charge, or the Medicare prevailing charge.

Confused? Most doctors are too. The Medicare explanation is that the physician's customary charge is what he normally bills most of his patients for a given service as indicated in the fee profile that the Medicare office maintains. The Medicare prevailing charge is set every July 1 at 75 percent of the customary charges made in the preceding calendar year by that physician and his colleagues in the same geographic region. The local Medicare "carrier," which may be an insurance company or Blue Shield-Blue Cross plan, and which pays doctors' bills, maintains a file of fee profiles and prevailing charge levels.

Partly because of this confusing method of setting fees, and partly because many doctors believe the payment of a medical bill is the patient's responsibility, many doctors will not accept Medicare reimbursement directly for the care of their elderly patients. Instead they request that the patient pay the bill directly and then get reimbursed by the Medicare carrier. That really means that the patient, instead of paying 20 percent of the doctor's fee, may pay as much as 40 or 50 percent. For example, if the physician charges twenty dollars for an electrocardiogram and interpretation, Medicare will only pay twelve dollars (75 percent of the *previous year's* customary charges of fifteen dollars). The patient then must pay the full twenty dollars, but receives only twelve dollars, or 60 percent, back from Medicare.

Under Medicaid this cannot happen to the patient, since payments are made directly to physicians, who must agree to accept the fee schedule of Medicaid as payment in full. Medicaid payments are generally limited to the lowest of (1) the doctor's actual charge for a service, (2) the median of his charge for a given service, derived from claims processed during the preceding year, and (3) the reasonable charge determined by Medicare. But in many cases, the state may reduce the fee even more, so that some doctor seeing Medicaid patients are accepting half or even a third of their usual fee for these patients. (For doctors this poses a real dilemma: They used to feel comfortable seeing charity patients for nothing; now that the government is paying, they are reluctant to see some patients at half the price they are charging others.)

4. *What to ask the doctor.* If you are covered by Medicare, first ask your doctor if he will accept "assignment," which means that he will accept whatever Medicare pays as 80 percent of his full fee, and charge only the additional 20 percent (after you have paid the deductible amount). Since many doctors today will not accept assignment, except perhaps in the case of a death (in which case the doctor gets paid more quickly that way), there are certain steps you can take to make certain that you get all the information needed to collect your reimbursement from the Medicare office:

Ask the doctor to fill out the medical part of the Medicare form, which he should have available in the office. Make sure the doctor or his office aide writes out the diagnosis on the form.

Make sure you get two copies of a fully itemized bill. One copy should be saved for your own records; the other should be attached to the Medicare form, and sent to the local Medicare processing office. The doctor's office can give you the address. If the bill lists other dates and services for which claims have already been submitted, cross these out.

If you don't receive your reimbursement or are asked for more information, or are confused by the "explanation of medical benefits" notice which you receive from Medicare, ask your doctor, his aide, or the Medicare carrier for assistance. The doctor's office will not receive copies of these communications from the Medicare office, so make sure to take your copies along with you.

5. *Supplemental insurance.* Medicare benefits are limited, both in the hospital and in nursing-home care, and a lengthy illness could easily wipe out any reserves that you or your family might have. It's advisable to purchase supplementary insurance from Blue Cross-Blue Shield or a commercial insurance carrier, which, like major-medical insurance, is especially tailored to give you more complete coverage (see previous chapter).

6. *How to find a Medicare or Medicaid doctor.* In a recent survey, 93 percent of doctors polled said they now take care of Medicare patients. But—if your financial situation is tight, you will have more trouble finding a doctor who will accept Medicare "assignment," in order to keep additional payments low. Only about 50 percent of doctors accept assignment, regularly or occasionally.

Even though the purpose of the Medicaid legislation is to provide health care without financial barriers, it may be difficult to find a doctor to provide the care. Many private practitioners do not want to see Medicaid patients, not only because of the low level of fees but also because of the difficulty in collecting from the state Medicaid office. Sometimes a doctor has to wait six months or so to have his bill paid. Because of very low fees, some doctors and hospitals have been accused of increasing the number of services for which they submit a bill, or billing Medicaid for unperformed laboratory services, in order to increase their income.

Most commonly, hospital outpatient departments will take care of Medicaid patients. In many cities, shared health facilities, sometimes called Medicaid "mills," exist. These medical groups consist of several physicians who rent space and primarily see Medicaid patients. Their care is often as good as that in a hospital outpatient department, but usually the time spent per patient is much less than would be the case in most private practitioners' offices. Your local welfare office can identify the physicians or groups in your area who take Medicaid patients.

7. *Where to turn for help with a disputed claim.* The Medicare program is administered nationally through carriers, which handle doctors' bills, and through "fiscal intermediaries," which handle hospital bills. These may be insurance companies or Blue Cross-Blue Shield plans. In each area of the country, the local carrier or intermediary is responsible for processing the claims submitted by Medicare patients for their doctors or hospitals. The handling of these claims does vary from one area to another, and it is frequently difficult for a patient to get a clear explanation of why a claim is denied or full reimbursement is not given. The first step is to go back to the Medicare carrier or intermediary with a written question, followed up by a phone call. If no satisfaction is obtained, consult your doctor or hospital. They can enlist the aid of the local medical society to contact the insurance office, determine the facts, and arrive at a decision.

8. *Where to find out more.* The best place to turn for help on Medicare coverage and problems of a general nature is the local Social Security office, which is listed in your phone book. (Request a copy of "Your Medicare Handbook.") The local welfare office should provide the same information regarding Medicaid. But be prepared to be persistent to get the information you want. You have a right to know what health coverage the government does provide for you and your family, and to have that information given to you promptly and clearly. If you encounter obstacles in getting the information from the Social Security or welfare office, the next best bet is to contact your local U.S. congressman or state representative. Their offices can get help for you.

25

HOW CAN YOU TELL IF THE DOCTOR'S BILL IS FAIR?

IF YOU HAD A PERSISTENT, GNAWING PAIN IN YOUR ABDOMEN, and you decided, one day in 1977, to visit a specialist in internal medicine in San Francisco or Los Angeles, chances are his fee for the visit alone, without lab tests or X rays, might have run as high as fifty dollars. Had you lived instead in Yoncalla, Oregon, and visited Dr. Lydia Emery, a fabled country doctor, her fee would have been the same as it was in 1949—one dollar for a visit in a cozy corner of her home-office. The time devoted by each physician to a history and physical examination might have been the same; the quality of the examination might have been similar, and the diagnosis might have been identical. But the fee would have been very different. Was either bill fair? Were both?

This example illustrates that the ground rules for charging for medical services are frequently obscure, even to the physicians who charge the fees. There are widespread discrepancies by specialty and by region of country between fees charged for the same service. According to a survey by *Medical Economics* magazine, in 1977 the median fee for a first office visit to a family physician in the Midwest was $10; for a family physician in the Far West, $16; for an internist in the South, $20; and for an obstetrician in the East, $25. The range of fees nationwide for internists for a first office visit showed that 5 percent charged $10, while 7 percent charged $50 or more, and about half charged $15–$20. The median fee nationally for complete obstetrical care by an obstetrician was $425, while for a family physician it was $300. The range showed that 17 percent of obstetricians charged $600 or more; 15 percent of the family physicians charged $225 or less. The range for surgical fees is just as widespread. The median fee nationally for an appendectomy was $325, but 6 percent of general surgeons charged $200 or less, while 18 percent charged $450 or more. Even more startling, obstetricians on the average charge $27 more for a dilatation and curettage if the purpose is abortion rather than diagnosis.

For the most part, charges for medical services are still set on the traditional fee-for-service basis by practicing physicians in each area of the country. Private patients without insurance coverage pay the doctor's usual fee. If a patient has private health-insurance coverage, the insurance customarily will pick up part of the usual fee and the patient will pay the balance. Under many Blue Shield policies, the doctor may be obligated through a participation agreement to accept what Blue Shield pays as full payment. The same is true under Medicaid. Under Medicare, the doctor may accept a Medicare fee schedule or set his own; either way, the patient pays part of the fee.

The federal government's campaign to encourage Health Maintenance Organizations (see Chapter 23) seeks to move physicians toward a prepaid type of practice in which a stipulated amount is paid per patient or per family each year for all medical attention, regardless of how much or how little is given. People who are members of HMOs need not concern themselves with whether the doctor's bill is fair, because they never see a bill for service, but only with whether the overall annual charge for membership is reasonable.

The concern about fair fees is heightened by the fact that physicians' fees rose at a faster average rate during the period 1966–1976 than all services and items in the Consumer Price Index. (During this same time, physicians' fees increased at a significantly lower rate than did hospital service charges.) Though health insurance covers much more of the average person's medical bills than was the case ten years ago, the actual out-of-pocket cost is just about the same, because fees and other medical charges have risen so rapidly.

How do doctors set their fees? Doctors talk to other doctors in the community to see what they charge for an office call, a house call, or a hospital call. In addition, physicians consult a number of fee schedules—from Blue Shield, Medicare, workman's compensation, or a state agency.

If a fee schedule appears too high or too low in relation to what other doctors are charging in the community, a physician may simply adjust it accordingly. Except for those in large group practices, doctors usually do not do cost accounting, and therefore do not set their fees in direct relation to the cost of providing services. But the increasing costs of rents, utilities, and office salaries do act as stimuli to fee increases.

One common approach to fee setting, called the Robin Hood concept, is fast disappearing. Doctors frequently would charge according to ability to pay, treating poor patients for practically nothing and making up the difference from their well-to-do patients. With increased coverage from Medicare, Medicaid, and other government programs for the indigent, doctors have tended to apply the same fees across the board. In fact, doctors new to a community are very conscious of what their Medicare fee profile will look like when first setting up a fee schedule. If fees are low to start, they become difficult to increase later. The profile determines what Medicare will pay for some time to come.

Charging what the traffic will bear also is on the wane, but at a less rapid rate. The demand for physician services in general exceeds the supply; even when it does not, increases in fees generally meet with little resistance on the part of the patients. Resistance is coming, however, from health insurers and the government. Government programs such as Medicare and Medicaid have set fee ceilings in some cases, or have frozen the fees of individual physicians at levels of one or two years ago. (This does not prevent the physician from charging private patients more than he can collect for his Medicaid patients.)

In a medical-center community there may be three or four levels of fees: one for the super-specialist who may head a medical-school department, a second for the practicing specialist in the community, a third for the family physician, and a fourth for the paramedical person (nurse, therapist, or physician's assistant) who may perform the service under the direction of the physician.

There is a strong argument that charges should remain the same for a given service no matter who performs it. For example, many physicians believe that the charge for a well-baby checkup should be the same whether the nurse or the physician sees the baby and mother. Other physicians feel just as strongly that there should be a differentiation in the charge, depending upon who renders the service. Organized medicine is resisting efforts by independent health practitioners (non-M.D.'s) to receive equal fees from government health-care financing programs. In theory, if a service is well performed—whether it is a well-baby checkup or open-heart surgery—the service should be worth the same to the patient. In practice, the patient may feel it is worth paying more for judgment, experience, and reputation—especially for a highly trained specialist.

In fact, in most areas of the country, a specialist will collect a higher fee for what is presumably the same procedure than will a family physician. Internists, for example, argue that they are entitled to higher fees for internal-medicine services than are general practitioners or family physicians. A South Carolina internist, Dr. C. Wallace Harper, argues that to give the same fee to any physician for a service would essentially "disenfranchise many excellent physicians who have spent arduous years of costly disciplined time and effort to achieve their skills, . . . would reward volume medicine at the expense of established and recognized quality care provided by qualified internists . . . and would provide a deterrent to the future recruitment of internists in rural areas." Dr. Harper's agument that internists are better qualifield to deal with certain difficult medical problems may be accepted by some family physicians, but they rebel against the idea that routine office visits should command a higher fee. So far, however, the fee differentiation by specialty has prevailed. Again, pressure by Medicare and Medicaid for negotiated fees based on services only, not on specialty, may charge the pattern.

Fees also vary between two nearby communities. For example, a surgeon's fee for a prostatectomy may be 20 percent less in the New York borough of Queens than in neighboring Manhattan, only a twenty-minute subway ride away. These variations can reflect the economic level in each community, overhead expenses, supply and demand related to physicians' services, and the historical pattern of fees in a community. Probably the latter is the most significant.

The nature of the services rendered is a major factor in fee setting. In most surgical procedures and obstetrics, the fee is for a package of services, regardless of how much or how little time is involved on the part of the physician. The package generally includes preoperative or postnatal care.

In the case of most medical care, the fee is based primarily on time spent by the physician. Historically, physicians have been paid less for thinking than for doing, and fees in the United States are still so structured. Internists, pediatricians, and family physicians frequently believe they are relatively underpaid when compared with specialists such as surgeons or radiologists, when their total efforts are matched. Some fee schedules attempt to recognize the time factor by paying more for a comprehensive physical exam than for a routine office visit, or paying more for a hospital visit related to intensive care than for a follow-up hospital visit to someone who is ready for discharge.

But time alone is not an adequate determinant of fees. Some physicians may be equally skilled, but unable to perform at the same rate of speed. Time spent on a seriously ill patient with a complex medical problem may be identical in quantity but not in quality to time spent treating a minor illness in a patient who is very talkative and complaining. A patient may feel that a physician's fee of fifty dollars for five minutes of time is excessive, even though the physician in that short time made an accurate diagnosis that relieved the patient's anxiety or led to a speedy cure. On the other hand, a physician who spends half an hour with a patient discussing a problem with a teenage daughter may feel he should receive fifty dollars for his time, even though the patient may think of this as a routine ten-dollar office visit.

The fee for laboratory and X-ray services usually covers a package including preparation for the test (drawing blood or setting up the patient on the X-ray table), for the test itself, and for interpretation of the test by the physician. However, many laboratory services are now performed outside the physician's office and there is a move underway to separate the fee into technical and professional components. In New York State, for example, the law now requires that an independent laboratory bill the patient directly for its charge in performing the laboratory test. The physician in turn must bill separately for his time spent in collecting the laboratory specimen and in interpreting the test results.

In 1956, the California Medical Association introduced a concept known as Relative Value Studies to help bring some order out of this chaotic approach to fee setting. Initially, the concept sought to relate the value of every medical service to the value of one standard office visit. For example, a standard office visit was given a unit value of 1, a house call might be given 1.5, and an X ray 2. Surgical procedures had a similar scale. Fees for different procedures could be determined by first selecting a dollar value for an office visit—say ten dollars—then multiplying by the number of units assigned in the Relative Value Studies.

Over the years, the Relative Value Studies have been changed to identify certain services more precisely, and to avoid unfair fee comparisons among the various types of services performed—i.e., between medicine and surgery or radiology. This basic approach has achieved a moderate degree of success. Some doctors in almost every state utilized it, as did many insurance carriers and government agencies. But in 1977, the Federal Trade Commission attacked the use of Relative Value Studies as price fixing and in restraint of trade. Their future is now highly questionable, even though the concept certainly helped eliminate some of the inequities in medical fees.

Now that you have some idea of the complexity of the fee-setting process, with its variations around the country, you can see how difficult it is to determine whether or not a given fee is fair.

Government agencies and health insurers compare an individual doctor's fees for the same service from one month to the next, and compare his fees with those charged by physicians of similar training and experience within the same area. This would be an impossible job for an individual patient.

Your best approach is to discuss fees in advance. You can ask the doctor's receptionist about his fees when you call for an appointment: What is his standard charge for a routine office visit, for a periodic health examination, or for some other standard procedure? In the case of an ophthalmologist, it might be a refraction test for glasses; in the case of a general surgeon, it might be an appendectomy.

If the receptionist suggests that you discuss fees with the doctor, then feel free to ask him the same question early in your first visit. If he hedges or becomes annoyed, you might want to consider another physician. Any doctor in private practice should be willing to discuss his charges openly and specifically.

The American Medical Association has long recommended that doctors do discuss services and fees frankly with patients. More recently, the AMA has recommended that physicians *initiate* a dialogue by volunteering fee information to patients in order to ease the patient's apprehension. It is suggested that such information cover a general range of fees and discuss different procedures such as lab tests, office billing procedures, arrangements for payment plans over time, and so forth.

In addition, physicians should be distributing information booklets covering fees, office hours, and a description of other services to patients in the waiting room. Some practices do this—but not enough.

Once you get the information from your doctor, what can you compare it with? Your basic consideration would be how his fee compares with that of other doctors with similar qualifications in your community. One way to determine this is to call the offices of two or three other physicians with similar practices, or group practices that provide similar services. If you ask about fees for two or three specific procedures, you can generally get a good idea of variations. If you are dealing with a family physician or an internist, ask about the fee for a routine office visit, an electrocardiogram, and the initial visit for hospital care. If you call a pediatrician or family physician, ask about the fee for care of a newborn infant and for a routine office visit. If you call a surgeon, check the fee for an appendectomy and a total hysterectomy (be sure to say "total," because there are different types). For an obstetrician, check on complete obstetrical care and total hysterectomy.

In a few areas of the country, physician directories have been published by consumer groups, listing physicians by specialty and by fees. For the most part, physicians have resisted this type of publication, although more recently the rules banning professional advertising have been lifted and some physicians may begin to advertise, including listing of fees. Medical societies are still cool to such listings.

However, county or state medical societies may sometimes be sources of fee information for the area, based on fee schedules provided by Medicare or state agencies. Local Blue Shield plans may also have published fee schedules available for comparison by consumers. And, of course, friends and relatives are *sometimes* a reliable source of information. Caution: Do not judge by Medicaid fee schedules, which in many states are as low as 33 percent of physicians' usual fees.

If your family doctor refers you to a specialist for surgery or other treatment, do not hesitate to ask your own doctor about the specialist's fees before going to see him. He can give you a good idea whether they are likely to be in line with those of other doctors with similar qualifications.

But do not stop there. Check with the specialist, too, when you first see him. If he quotes you a figure higher than that suggested by your family doctor, consult your family doctor and let him assist in any negotiations if necessary.

26

WHAT YOU SHOULD KNOW ABOUT HOSPITAL AND NURSING-HOME CHARGES

BILL AND MARTHA WILLIAMS HAD A DIFFICULT AUTUMN. First their three-year-old, Kevin, who had had a chronic ear infection, entered one of New York City's finest university hospitals for what was described as simple one-day surgery to drain the ear, to remove the adenoids, and to insert a plastic tube in the ear to keep it open. Kevin entered the hospital at seven in the morning and was home again by eight that evening for an uneventful recovery.

Two months later his infant brother, Tom, only six weeks old, was running a very high fever and showed signs of con- vulsions. The pediatrician rushed him directly from his office to the hospital, where he remained in an isolation unit from Monday until Friday, being treated with antibiotics after numerous spinal taps and other tests to determine whether he had spinal meningitis. The verdict fortunately was nega- tive, and Tom returned home to join his brother, once again in good health.

The Williamses, pleased that modern medical science had treated both children so well in the hospital, were less than pleased with the hospital bills they received. The first, from the major university hospital, was for almost eight hundred dollars for the one-day stay, including the use of the operating room and various tests, plus items that just did not make sense to the parents. By comparison, the stay at a local communiy hospital for the baby, Tom, was priced at little more than six hundred dollars for almost five days of care. In both cases, Mr. Williams' health insurance covered most of the costs, but he was more than mildly curious as to how hospitals could come up with such different rates.

In the case of the bills for the care of the two Williams boys, the difference in the location of the hospitals and the types of special services required apparently made the difference. Hospitals in the same geographic area vary widely in the rates charged for rooms and for special or "ancillary" services. The semiprivate-room rate at a major university hospital may be as much as three to four hundred dollars a day, while a community hospital in the suburbs of the same city might charge only eighty to one hundred twenty-five dollars a day.

The rationale is that the patient in the university hospital has available all the sophisticated services and personnel needed to provide instantaneous life support in any emergency, whereas the community hospital is equipped to deal with more routine surgical, medical, and obstetrical cases. The university hospital is certain to have a large staff of interns and residents (physicians in training), a portion of whose salaries come from the services they perform as part of the hospital staff. In the community hospital, doctors' fees are paid only to the attending physician who practices in the community, and are not added to the hospital bill.

Hospitals as a group have had a much higher rate of increase in costs than any other component of the health-care cost index. In the year 1977, the rate of increase in hospital expenditures was 15.6 percent. In 1977, the cost for an average patient-day varied from slightly over one hundred dollars in a small hospital with less than one hundred beds to over four hundred dollars for a metropolitan university hospital with five hundred beds or more.

Some people think that a hospital is run pretty much as a hotel, with room services, meals, and a few other niceties thrown in. That is no longer true. Major items of hospital costs include the building, equipment, personnel, and particularly specialty services that may be used only occasionally, yet account for a high percentage of cost just to be available. Each of us is paying for the availability of new life-prolonging and lifesaving equipment and services every time we enter the hospital.

It is estimated that new medical technologies directly or indirectly account for almost 50 percent of the increase in hospital costs since 1950. Hospitals need highly specialized personnel to operate these pieces of equipment. One example of this is the growth of coronary-care units with specialized monitoring equipment to keep heart-attack victims alive longer. Another example is the new computerized tomography scanners, which may cost the hospital over five hundred thousand dollars each; while these scanners are extremely useful in detecting brain tumors or other problems much earlier than might be done otherwise, the costs of acquiring and operating them are astronomic. In the period from 1971 to 1973 alone, there was a 96-percent increase in the number of hospitals that offered radioisotope facilities and a 60-percent increase in those that offered psychiatric facilities.

Laboratory testing has become more common, and more sophisticated as well. Costs of supplies and personnel have gone up, and so have the number of tests. The same is true of X-ray examinations. Increased utilization of both lab and X-ray services alone added an average of thirty-one dollars to a patient's bill in the space of less than five years. Because such equipment is getting more sophisticated, fewer physicians have the necessary lab and X-ray equipment in their offices; instead, they refer the work to hospitals.

Another factor that enters into current high hospital

charges is that the new technology is not only costly to perform, but costly to follow up. Patients requiring intensive care, organ transplants, fetal monitoring, or open-heart surgery may have many complications that require longer stays and closer monitoring in the hospital. Beyond that, all the new drugs available in the past twenty years have led to a higher percentage of adverse reactions, which now account for as many as one in twenty hospital admissions.

The cost of labor in hospitals has risen dramatically, too. Hospital employees used to be underpaid compared with most of industry, but now not only do we have more employees—3.4 per patient compared with 2.3 per patient fifteen years earlier—but bringing their wage rates up has accounted for 37 percent of the increase in hospital costs. Hospital workers are now earning a little more than the average for nonfarm workers, and their wage rates continue to rise faster than those of other workers. Finally, professional liability premiums, to protect hospitals and physicians against the costs of malpractice suits, have increased an average of 30 cents annually per patient visit. Hidden costs to protect against malpractice suits include an increased number of laboratory and X-ray tests that are done as part of "defensive medicine."

Hospital charges start with a detailed cost-accounting system, but the cost-accounting system does not mean much in terms of what the hospital charges are. For the most part, hospitals are paid different rates by Blue Cross plans, by commercial insurance carriers, by uninsured individuals, by Medicare, by Medicaid, and by Health Maintenance Organization programs. In many cases, the government-run programs pay the least for hospital services; Blue Cross programs pay somewhat more, and patients covered by commercial health insurance or those who are uninsured pay a higher total rate than everyone else. There is no question that the system is unfair, even though paying agencies and state regulatory bodies perpetuate it.

If you think the subject of hospital costs is confusing to

you, remember that it is also confusing to your physician, who does not normally get involved in pricing, or in billing for hospital care. In fact, Russell B. Roth, M.D., a Pennsylvania urologist, did a study several years ago to determine whether practicing physicians were familiar with the hospital charges for goods and services that they order for their patients. His study showed that only 13 percent of the responses were accurate, 41 percent were too high, and 45 percent were too low. He noted that the general tendency of physicians was "to underestimate the cost of goods and services . . . by an average of 17 percent."

To illustrate how a typical hospital identifies its sources of revenue from patient services, let us look at this review of a typical 200-bed community hospital as developed by W. R. Friedman, Jr., a health-care financial analyst. In this hospital, 45 percent of the revenue comes from what are defined as routine services: room and board, administration, general maintenance such as housekeeping and laundry, food, plant operation, and medical records. Another 44 percent of the revenue comes from ancillary services: laboratory, radiology, pharmacy, operating room, electrocardiology, anesthesia, intravenous solutions, and inhalation therapy. The emergency room and other outpatient services account for 11 percent of revenue, a fast-growing area because of the shortage of primary physicians in most communities.

In the same hospital, 35 percent of the income is paid by Medicare, another 35 percent by Blue Cross, 15 percent by Medicaid, and the other 15 percent by commercial insurance and individual payments. Only in the latter category are the full charges of the hospital paid. In specialty hospitals, particularly psychiatric hospitals, insurance pays a lower percentage of income.

Because of the complexity of hospital costs and charging systems, it is not likely that you can modify your bill to any great extent unless you believe that the care was inadequate or that the hospital made mistakes for which it should be held responsible. However, it is an excellent idea to ask the hospital for a copy of your full bill and to check each item to make sure that no charges were duplicated. It is also an excellent idea to review the bill with your physician and your health insurance agent.

State hospital commissions have unsuccessfully attempted to monitor and control hospital costs. In the past year or so, President Carter and Congress have debated proposals for hospital-cost containment. The voluntary organizations— American Hospital Association, Federation of American Hospitals, and American Medical Association—are urging voluntary efforts by their members to hold down the cost spiral. Nothing has worked yet.

What about nursing-home costs? Basic charges in nursing homes vary much more widely than hospital charges, even when the homes are in the same general area. Charges depend upon the following factors:

Geographic location
Quality and type of home
Number and range of services rendered
Size of the staff in relation to the patient population
Quality of the services rendered
Professional and technical status of the staff
Size of the home
Rate of occupancy
Nutritional standards
Recreational and other facilities available
Characteristics of the patient population and degree of
 care necessary
Type of accommodation used
Source of payment for care

Around the country, average costs per patient-day can vary as much as 100 percent, say from New Mexico to Illinois. Even within one state the range can be as great. Charges are generally highest in the Northeast and West, lower in the North Central region, and lowest in the South.

Charges generally run higher in proprietary (for-profit)

homes than in nonprofit homes, or if not, services are skimpier. Charges also generally increase with the amount of care received, and with the level of nursing supervision. Larger homes tend to give higher charges than smaller ones, probably because they offer more services.

Because there is no uniformity in the way nursing homes make their charges, it is important to bear in mind the following:

1. Skilled nursing homes normally provide different classes of accommodations (private, semiprivate, and ward) and charges normally vary by class of accommodation.

2. For private-pay patients (nonwelfare), the nursing home normally makes charges for ancillary services (drugs, physical therapy, laboratory, X ray, etc.).

3. Some nursing homes vary their charges depending upon the amount of nursing care required by the patient (who may be incontinent, in need of hand feeding, etc.).

27

WHAT TO DO IF YOU'RE
DISSATISFIED ABOUT A BILL

A HEADLINE IN A LOS ANGELES NEWSPAPER A COUPLE OF YEARS ago read: "Popcorn removed from ear of child—bill totals $420."

The father of a three-year-old complained that the doctor simply plucked a piece of popcorn out of his daughter's ear with a pair of tweezers. "I think I was taken," he said.

Variations of that story are repeated daily in towns and cities all over the country. In this case, the child's family doctor had tried to remove the popcorn unsuccessfully and then had sent the child to a specialist; he put her in the hospital and removed the popcorn under general anesthesia. The child's hearing was unimpaired—but not her father's pocketbook. He paid the hospital $259, the family doctor $11, the ear, nose, and throat specialist $100, and the hospital anesthesiologist $51.

The child's father, dissatisfied with both doctors' and hospital bills, took his case to the public by calling a newspaper. He received plenty of publicity, as did the doctors and the hospital, but he was unable to reduce the bills by so much as a nickel. In general, a public cry of anguish is seldom likely to result in settlement of what might be a legitimate complaint.

Here is an approach that has a better chance of success:

1. Use an ounce of prevention. Find out in advance from the doctor and the hospital what the charges are likely to be. (See chapters 24 and 25.)

2. If a doctor's bill seems excessive, call him up and ask him to explain the charges. If his secretary doesn't want to put you through to the doctor, tell her what the question is and request that the doctor call you back. Make it clear, however, that you do expect to talk with the doctor about the bill—not simply with his secretary or bookkeeper. He may not have set the charge, but he is by far the best person to reduce it.

3. If the doctor refuses to adjust his charge, and you are not satisfied with his explanation, tell him that you would like to have the matter reviewed by the local medical society and ask him to give you the name of the person to contact there. If he fails to do so, look up your county medical society in the phone book (usually listed under the name of the county) and tell the person who answers your call that you wish to register a complaint about a doctor's bill.

4. You will be put in touch with the chairman of the local grievance committee. He will probably ask you to present your complaint in writing, and perhaps to appear before the committee. Make sure to tell him that you already have discussed the problem with the doctor but have not been satisfied with his response. The committee will then review your complaint, comparing the charge and the services rendered with the "usual and customary" fees for similar services in the area.

The committee also may discuss your complaint with the doctor, and then will let you know its recommendations. If the committee recommends a reduced fee, the doctor is not bound by this decision (whether or not he is a member of the medical society); but most doctors are likely to accept such a recommendation.

5. If the doctor refuses to go along with the recommenda-

tion of a reduced fee, or if the committee feels the fee is fair but you still do not, take your complaint to your state board of medical examiners, which may have an office to deal with fee problems. Otherwise, consult a lawyer before paying the bill. He can advise you about the chances of success in a possible court challenge—a safer procedure than making your own decision not to pay the bill and ending with a court order to pay, plus the expenses of a trial.

6. If you feel that you have been overcharged by a specialist to whom you were referred by another physician, consult your referring doctor before going to the medical-society grievance committee. Frequently a family doctor can gain the cooperation of a specialist. After all, the latter is dependent upon the former's goodwill for referrals.

Will a similar procedure work for a hospital bill that seems too high? Unfortunately, the chances are practically nil that you can gain a reduction, unless you can demonstrate that you were billed for services not rendered. (It does happen that hospitals mix up patient charges for drugs, lab services, etc., so it's worth checking the bill item by item.)

Every hospital has its standard schedule of charges for room and board, laboratory and other diagnostic tests, use of operating rooms, and special services. Most of these rates have been accepted by Blue Cross, Medicare, and other insuring agencies as a basis for payment. An individual patient is unlikely to change any such established charges. Even if he feels that unnecessary laboratory or X-ray services were performed, he has little recourse. The hospital will insist that the tests were ordered by the doctor, and the doctor will respond that he has been following standard hospital admission practices in ordering such tests.

The patient's best recourse against hospital overcharging is to have adequate health insurance and let the insurance company fight his battles. As a long shot, you can register a complaint with the local hospital administrator and ask what can be done to reduce the hospital charge. If his response is inadequate, forward your complaint to the state hospital association. (Your local hospital can give you the address.)

Perhaps the public forum of a newspaper may be a useful last resort to awaken the community to excessive charges by doctors and hospitals—even though it won't put any money back in your pocket. The episode of the child with popcorn in her ear focused public attention on the hospital and doctors concerned. What's more, it led to professional attention through an article in *Medical Economics* magazine. A poll of its readers indicated that many physicians felt the charges were excessive—primarily because the doctors were overcautious in hospitalizing the child for two nights and ordering more tests than might be necessary.

WHAT TO DO ABOUT RISING
HEALTH-CARE COSTS

TWO SURGICAL RESIDENTS AT A BIG DENVER HOSPITAL WERE asked to review bills on some of the patients they had seen in recent weeks. They looked at the record of Stanley Marshall, a fifty-five-year-old construction worker who had been admitted complaining of abdominal pain, which they believed to be caused by an ulcer. Surgery was performed, but the surgeons missed a perforation or small hole in the duodenum, part of the intestine, which led to five months of additional hospitalization for Mr. Marshall. The residents were staggered by the $45,000 hospital bill. If it accomplished nothing else, it made them very acutely aware of the economic implications of errors in clinical care.

In this hospital, physicians on the staff, residents, and students attend a conference each week to discuss the economics of care and discover ways of reducing costs that are consistent with good medical care. Sometimes the findings are much less dramatic than the $45,000 bill. For example, one student discovered that an electrocardiogram and laboratory work on blood had been performed in the emergency department on one patient and then repeated only an hour later when the patient had been admitted upstairs to the hospital bed. Extra cost: $45. In another case, a hospital bill showed that one test to determine the level of blood gases had been repeated needlessly three times in a morning, at a cost of $30 each.

According to Dr. Ben Eiseman, a surgeon at the Denver hospital, "the shopping list is endless and enormously expensive. When a particular physician seems unconcerned about needless procedures, and the expenses involved, it is occasionally suggested facetiously that perhaps this amount should be deducted from his paycheck. This seems to carry the message."

Medical-care costs continue to grow faster than inflation, and even though third parties, or health-insurance agencies, pay most of the costs of care, Americans as taxpayers and employees and purchasers of goods and services are really paying for those increased costs. Hospital charges have risen even faster than physicians' fees, and the government is anxiously looking for ways to control or stem the rise of costs. Not only do federal government costs keep going up, but state government costs keep going up because of the increased costs of Medicaid. New York State alone spent more than $15 billion for overall health-care costs in 1976, more than double the amount spent in 1969. Even though government programs are paying more and more of the bill, the direct payments by individuals continue to increase. Those sixty-five and over, who can least afford it, are paying almost double out-of-pocket compared with ten years ago.

Can you do anything to control hospital costs? You cannot do much to control overall costs; but you can do something to control the cost of an individual hospital stay.

Some of the savings keep money in your own pocket, even though private or government insurers are paying most of the bill. Indirectly, any reduction that you can make in hospital costs may save you money in future insurance premiums or taxes.

You'll need your doctor's cooperation to achieve any substantial savings. On your own, you may be able to save a few dollars by selecting semiprivate rather than private accommodations, or doing without a television or telephone, if you have a choice. But the really substantial savings will come only if you and your doctor can shorten your stay in the hospital or eliminate some borderline expenses.

Here is a checklist of possible savings to review with your physician.

1. If you are having elective surgery, such as a hernia operation, a hysterectomy, or a prostate removal, have as much of the preoperative work as possible completed before you are admitted to the hospital as a bed patient. Most hospitals today are glad to have you come in a day or two before the operation for necessary lab tests, X rays, physical exams, etc., then go home to bed. Once the test results are in, and the doctor has you scheduled for surgery, you can enter the hospital the night before—or even early on the morning of the operation.

2. For any problem that isn't an emergency, the biggest waste of money is entering the hospital on a Friday. Very few hospital laboratories or X-ray departments work on anything but an emergency basis over the weekend. Chances are, all you would get is a good rest (if you call being awakened at six in the morning for breakfast a good rest). The doctor can't really get the information he needs to start treatment until these diagnostic facilities open up on Monday.

3. Encourage your doctor to schedule all your diagnostic tests in as short a time as possible. Frequently, a hospital may take blood tests today, X rays tomorrow, and then remember that a urine sample was never collected. Three days of waiting around for the test results may not bother your doctor, but they can be frustrating and costly to you and your health-insurance company.

4. Private-duty nursing may be a borderline expense that comes out of your own pocket, because many insurance plans do not cover this cost. The doctor may order private nurses because he feels you won't get sufficiently close attention from the floor nurses during a period of acute illness

or immediately after surgery. Sometimes it's possible to have a close relative stay at the bedside, and simply alert the floor nurse to immediate needs. This can save fifty dollars or more just for one eight-hour shift.

5. Get out of the hospital as soon as possible. Even though you may still need some nursing care, physical therapy, and rest, almost any alternative will be cheaper than the hospital. These include moving to an extended-care facility, to a nursing home, or to your own home under some type of home-care program.

Any of these alternatives might well reduce the cost of care by 40 percent or more. This is a saving well worth the effort required from you and your doctor, even though you may need to revisit the hospital on an outpatient basis for an X ray, a lab test, or physical therapy.

6. Follow your doctor's advice rather than that of well-intentioned relatives or friends, who may urge you to extend your hospital stay and get a few extra days of rest. If the doctor feels you are ready to go home or to a facility offering less intensive care, take his advice. He is usually a better judge than you or your relatives as to whether you really require a full range of hospital services. In fact, disregarding his advice can be costly to your own pocket. Every hospital today has a utilization committee to review whether or not the length of a hospital stay is medically justified. If the committee decided that you could have left the hospital a few days earlier than you did, your insurance probably will not pay for those extra days. You may be stuck with the bill.

7. Discuss the course of your hospitalization in advance with your doctor. If he doesn't want to predict how long you will be in the hospital, ask what the average length of stay has been for patients with similar problems. There are national averages for length of stay by diagnosis, although these can vary by region of the country and by the condition and age of individual patients. If you are informed in this

way, you can better plan for an earlier discharge, home care, etc.

8. Talk with the hospital admissions office and/or cashier before entering the hospital if possible—or have a relative do so. Get a clear idea of the hospital's basic room charges, charges for extras, charges for special services, and billing practices. Know in advance whether or not the hospital charges extra for the operating room and recovery room, for tests ordered over the weekend, or for special diets. You'll avoid unwelcome surprises.

9. Find out if the hospital charges for its rooms by the full day, the half day, or the hour. In some cases you may save a few dollars simply by adjusting the exact time you enter or leave the hospital.

10. Find out whether the hospital is going to demand payment from you weekly, before discharge, or after discharge. Another question may come up at discharge time: Should you tip hospital nurses or other employees? As a rule, no. It's a nice gesture, however, to make a small gift that's appropriate for the nursing staff rather than any one individual.

Can you do anything to control nursing-home costs? You can do more yourself to achieve substantial savings in nursing-home costs than in hospital costs. The choice of a nursing home is much broader and you are not so dependent on the doctor's decision as you are when he puts you in the hospital. Here are ways to hold down the cost of nursing-home care:

1. Select the type of home that provides the specific level of care required. For example, some nursing homes, called extended care facilities, provide essentially the same quality and type of care that a hospital provides to convalescent patients. Unless this level of care is needed, you may be paying more than necessary. Similarly, a chronically ill patient who needs primarily custodial care shouldn't be paying for skilled nursing care.

2. Select a nursing home meeting the requirements of your health-insurance coverage. Otherwise you may have to pay most or all of the bill yourself. Under Medicare, for instance, a nursing home must be certified as a skilled-nursing-care facility before a patient can receive benefits. Private insurance policies vary considerably and you must check your policy to be sure what kind of nursing care, if any, is covered.

3. If a patient is convalescing, select a nursing home that emphasizes rehabilitative services. The cost per day may be slightly higher, but the real benefit comes from restoring a person to active functioning sooner. Rehabilitative services include physical therapy, occupational therapy, speech therapy, etc.

4. If a home health-care program is available in your area, consult with the doctor to see how rapidly the patient can be transferred from a nursing home to a home environment with skilled care.

5. If a person is likely to require custodial care for the rest of his life, consider one of the few church- or fraternal-group-sponsored homes that still offer a life-care contract for a lump-sum payment. With the rapidly rising cost of care, this type of contract may be a saving in the long run. At least, the amount of the payment is determined in advance, regardless of how long the patient may live.

Caution: Don't be penny-wise and pound-foolish. The quality of care at nursing homes varies even more widely than costs. Many nursing homes have failed to meet minimal standards of Medicare, Medicaid, and the American Nursing Home Association. So it's best to start by identifying those nursing homes that offer a reasonable level of care, and then to consider costs.

Can you do anything to control physician costs? Yes, you can, and this is the area to start, since it's through the physician that costs for hospital and nursing-home care are incurred. Here are some ideas that can be particularly helpful:

1. Avoid doctor-hopping. It's costly to go from one doctor to another, not only because of the extra office-visit fee, but because the tests ordered by the second physician frequently repeat those that have been performed previously. If in doubt about what your doctor is telling you, ask him to suggest a consultant and to provide the consultant with the results of your lab and X-ray tests and a summary of your record.

2. Don't use the doctor as a source of solace for every minor ailment. Most illnesses are self-limiting. If your ache, pain, or sore throat appears to be of a garden variety, wait a few days to see if the problem will clear up without a visit to the physician. Exceptions, of course, are injuries, foreign objects in the eye or ear, severe attacks of pain or bleeding.

3. Take careful note of what the doctor advises, whether in regard to medications, exercises, diet, or whatever therapy, and follow through on his advice so as to minimize repeat visits. The doctor frequently tells someone with an infection to take the medication for ten days whether he or she feels better or not. A person who fails to listen to this advice may feel better and stop taking the drug after three days. Result: The infection may recur in another week or two. That means another visit to the doctor!

4. When you call for an appointment with the doctor, tell his nurse what the problem is and ask if there is any specific information—or any specimens, such as urine or stool—that you should bring with you to save a repeat visit. Perhaps she will suggest not eating prior to the visit so that the doctor can take a sample of "fasting blood."

5. When the doctor prescribes a medication, check with him as to whether there are pharmacies which sell the drug at a lower cost than others, or ask him if there is an alternative therapy that is equally effective but less expensive.

6. Resist pressure from relatives who want you to visit the doctor—unless you yourself feel ill enough to do so. Resist the pressure of relatives who want you to enter the

hospital—unless you and your doctor feel this is the best course to pursue. Well-meaning relatives can push you into unnecessary medical care because of their uninformed concern.

7. Avoid entering a hospital for the purpose of tests. If it's at all possible, have the tests conducted on an outpatient basis. Sometimes the doctor may prefer, for his convenience, to see you in the hospital for two or three days for various X rays or laboratory tests. You might be able to obtain these at lower cost and without any greater inconvenience by going to the hospital clinic, to a radiologist's office, or to a private laboratory where the tests can be performed and the results relayed to your physician.

8. Don't use the hospital emergency room unless you are unable to reach your regular physician. The hospital emergency room will usually be more costly for the initial visit, and may require repeating certain lab and X-ray tests that have already been performed at your doctor's office. In addition, the emergency room does not have the benefit of key information about you which is in the medical record in your physician's office and which takes time to collect again and analyze.

9. If you are embarking on a new type of therapy for a chronic disease or a serious problem, bring a close relative or friend to the doctor's office with you, to listen with you to his advice and to give you reinforcement as you begin to carry out the therapy recommended. A special family-and-patient education program in some clinics has reduced the revisits needed by patients with asthma or bleeding problems, because a family member was helping them with information and support during their illness.

10. Over the long run, the most important thing you can do to control medical costs is to change your life-style so as to reduce the risk of serious illness. This means stopping cigarette smoking, wearing your seat belts while driving, controlling your weight and eating a balanced diet,

drinking alcohol in moderation only, and exercising regularly.

As citizens, all of us can work toward improved life-styles that can do more to keep us healthy and control our health-care costs than all the doctors and hospitals put together. We can also support the efforts of voluntary and governmental agencies seeking to utilize our health-care resources as adequately as possible. For example, the administrator and the board of trustees of your community hospital may seek to add two hundred beds to the hospital's capacity. But this may be a waste of money if there are already enough or too many hospital beds in the area. Similarly, it may be more convenient to have cobalt-therapy equipment in a hospital only five minutes away, but if there is a similar unit in a hospital twenty-five minutes away, the second one really may not be needed. Health Systems Agencies, created by the federal government, seek to monitor use of resources on a local basis; citizen participation is mandated.

With cooperation by a combination of individuals, doctors, hospitals, and government officials, we can keep health-care costs within bounds. Without that kind of cooperation, even a national system of health insurance would not prevent health-care costs from taking more and more of our income each year, leaving us less and less for the good things of life.

29

CAN YOU REALLY MEASURE QUALITY OF MEDICAL CARE?

MOST OF THE CONTENT OF THIS BOOK IS DESIGNED TO HELP you get good-quality medical care and reduce the risk of getting poor care. But I have a confession to make: I do not know precisely how to define the quality of medical care. Furthermore, the experts I have consulted do not seem to be in agreement about how to measure the quality of medical care, or whether in fact it can be measured.

In a recent study, "Assessing Quality in Health Care: An Evaluation," prepared by the Institute of Medicine of the National Academy of Sciences, the authors wrote, "Most statements . . . refer to the need to ensure high quality medical care at reasonable cost, but do not include measurable objectives or methods for improving the quality of care. Indeed, the margin by which quality might be improved is not known. No program official [whom we interviewed] was able to offer even a rough estimate of the extent of deficient or inappropriate care. Without such a measure, it becomes difficult to determine whether a program is achieving its objectives."

One of the hospitals studied by the Institute was Overlook Hospital of Summit, New Jersey. Overlook reported successes with its quality assurance program. The program led to increased use of rehabilitation facilities for stroke patients, decrease in inappropriate kidney X rays performed on young patients, and almost 100-percent compliance by surgeons with criteria for hysterectomies. In the jargon used by medical-care-quality experts, these are what are known as "process" measurements. That is, certain specialists in each area decided that, in their opinion, care would be better if there were more rehabilitation services, fewer X rays, or tighter surgical criteria. Using *their* standards, the quality of care at Overlook Hospital was improved.

But can you, as a patient, be sure that the quality of care was improved because the process of care seemed better? Isn't the outcome of medical care the most important determinant of quality? It doesn't really matter, does it, whether drug A or drug B is used if the patient is discharged alive, feeling better, and able to function normally once again? There always seems to be more than one right way to get a job done—in medicine as well as in other areas of life. And from year to year, there are new approaches to diagnosis and treatment that make previous standards seem outmoded.

Outcome may be the answer that looks most important in assessing quality—but may be hard to define. Quality experts in San Joaquin, California, reported that an eighty-year-old man had been hospitalized repeatedly as a result of the side effects of medication he was taking. After each hospitalization he was in good shape and returned home—only to have the problem recur within three months. Finally, someone had a bright idea: Arrangements were made for a visiting nurse to supervise the old man's medications at home, and he was able to stay out of the hospital. In effect, a new resource was introduced—the use of a visiting nurse. Thus, the appropriate utilization of resources can be called a third method of measuring quality of care.

You notice that I have not mentioned patient satisfaction as a measurement of quality. While it definitely should be included, the trouble is that different people are satisfied with different results. Let's take the illustration of two people in their seventies, each with bad arthritis of the hip. Each had been walking with great difficulty and considerable pain. Eleanor Jones had one of the new hip-replacement operations, and in three months was walking almost free of pain and with only a slight limp. She used a cane to steady herself when she went out alone. She told her doctor that she was very pleased with the outcome of the surgery and that now she was planning a trip to Europe with a younger friend. Fred Newman, same age, had a similar operation two weeks after Eleanor's. His physical results were about the same. But when he saw his doctor for a checkup six months after surgery, he banged his cane on the doctor's desk and said, "I thought I would never have to use this damn thing again! You told me this operation would take care of all my arthritis—and it hasn't." What's quality to one person just isn't to another.

It should be easiest to use defined measurements of outcome as the best way to measure the quality of care, or at least so it seems. It should be possible to say that medical care should achieve certain specified results with a diabetic, a hypertensive, a person with stomach cancer, or a hay-fever sufferer. But it just doesn't work that way. No two persons are exactly alike, nor are two persons with the same disease likely to react the same way to the same therapy. Factors that make a difference include the patient's attitude, the patient's general state of health, the patient's family and their attitude and support, availability of financing, the clinical skills of the doctor, the medications he uses, the surgical or radiological support he calls on, the hospital facilities, and the nurses.

Direct intervention by doctors is only a part of the total picture that affects the outcome of illness for any person. For example, a review of patients with hip fractures at Overlook Hospital showed that more than 30 percent of the patients had decubitus ulcers (bed sores). Their hips were mending nicely, but complications were coming from just lying in bed. The hospital instituted a program to prevent and treat pressure sores, by hiring a special rehabilitation nurse.

Frequently the individual himself or herself is responsible for a bad outcome of illness. National studies show that about half the Americans who have been diagnosed as having high blood pressure are not following the treatment programs outlined for them. Nor are they coming back for checkups. Yet it is known that high blood pressure, if untreated, causes a much higher incidence of stroke, and therefore a shorter life-span. People with hypertension will have a poor outcome if not treated, yet they are blocking their own ability to get medical care.

The medical profession, hospitals, and the government have all been trying for years to do something about improving the quality of care. A good deal has been done already, despite the complexity of the problem. Here are some steps that have been taken:

1. State medical boards are taking a closer look than ever before at the competence of physicians who are practicing in their states. Licensing requirements are stiffer than they were twenty or thirty years ago, and many states are now moving to require that physicians provide at least minimal evidence that they are keeping up. So far, this evidence has mostly been in the form of acquired number of hours of continuing medical education—not a very valid measurement of the quality of care or of the competence of the physician—but at least some evidence that the doctor hasn't stayed in the dark ages. This is more than can be said of any other profession (with the exception of airline pilots, who are reexamined at least annually).

2. Medical specialty boards, such as in internal medicine, family practice, surgery, and obstetrics, offer certifying examinations once a young physician has completed his residency training in the specialty. Now the American Board of Family Practice has required that any specialist in family practice be recertified every six years on the basis of an examination, evidence of his continuing medical education,

and at least a brief review of some of the medical records of his patients. Other specialty boards are following suit; by the mid-1980's almost all of the twenty-two specialty boards will require periodic recertification of their members.

3. Hospitals, through their medical-staff bylaws, have imposed certain quality restrictions on physicians who use the hospital as their workshop. In order to get privileges to do surgery, deliver babies, or treat heart attacks, physicians must meet certain standards established by the medical staff of the hospital and approved by the board of trustees. These standards vary widely from hospital to hospital; occasionally a doctor will lose his privileges if he fails to meet the standards after several warnings. Hospitals uncommonly exercise such restrictions because doctors sometimes sue hospitals for depriving them of their "workshops" and doctors tend to look at errant colleagues with a "there-but-for-the-grace-of-God-go-I" attitude. Hospitals also have special committees to examine the results of surgical procedures to determine whether the surgery was necessary and whether in fact the organ removed was diseased. (These are called tissue committees.)

4. In 1951, a specialized organization, the Joint Commission on Accreditation of Hospitals, was formed by the American College of Surgeons, the American College of Physicians, the American Medical Association, and the American Hospital Association. The Joint Commission was charged with the responsibility of surveying hospitals around the country according to certain minimal standards, and either accrediting them, putting them on probation, or denying them accreditation. These standards were minimal to begin with, but have been substantially raised over the years, covering a variety of areas of housekeeping, cleanliness, fire standards, operating-room and emergency-room procedures, medical-staff procedures, nursing, etc. When Medicare and Medicaid programs were passed by Congress in 1966, new teeth were added to the hospital accreditation process. In fact, hospitals need to have accreditation in order to

receive payment under these government programs.

5. The newest pressure for quality review has come from 1972 federal legislation calling for the establishment of Professional Standards Review Organizations (PSROs). About two hundred such regional organizations have been created around the United States, for the most part through doctors living and practicing in each region. They are charged with the responsibility of monitoring the quality of care in all area hospitals. When deficiencies are identified, corrective-action programs are instituted.

One of the pioneers in medical-care evaluation, Richard E. Anonsen, M.D., a family physician in Minneapolis and a board member of the Foundation of Health Evaluation, describes a typical effort to improve quality in the hospitals in the Twin Cities area:

"If a patient with chest pain is admitted to a coronary-care unit, we want him to have electrocardiograms and enzyme studies; we want him to have oxygen and to go on a heart monitor. And we want justification for any medication. We don't say what medication or what enzyme studies. We know that in this community 85 percent of these patients will be discharged alive at fourteen to twenty-one days. So if we find a hospital that has a 30-percent mortality rate, we go to that institution to find out why.

"Maybe they don't even have a coronary-care unit. Or maybe several physicians using the hospital haven't kept up on this problem. Or maybe one doctor is deficient—he doesn't get out of bed and come down to take care of his patients. So we go to the staff and ask them to correct the situation—further education, better equipment, using a consultant, or whatever."

Under PSRO, physicians tend to rely heavily on record analysts who do a preliminary review of medical records and bring to the attention of a medical reviewer only those that show something outside the standards already set. For example, in one Utah hospital, a nurse coordinator noted that a patient with urinary-tract infection should have been prepared for discharge the next day, but hadn't been. She alerted the reviewing physician, then contacted the patient's own physician to find out why the patient wasn't being sent home. This kind of quality review can help people get well faster and at lower cost, if properly administered.

As a matter of fact, as this story illustrates, more care doesn't always mean better care. There is a definite relationship between length of stay, cost of stay, and quality of care for people. Henry E. Simmons, M.D., formerly director of the Office of Professional Standards Review of the U.S Department of Health, Education and Welfare, pointed out in 1975 that "there are some 375,000 cataract operations done each year in this country. The traditional length of stay for this operation is 5–8 days, with marked regional differences. Now there are about 7,000 cases in medical literature to show that you can do cataract surgery safely on an ambulatory basis [without staying the night in the hospital]. The profession simply has to say it is no longer necessary to hospitalize 5–8 days for cataract surgery. This could free up $250 million a year to be used elsewhere for medical care."

Changes in care that allow for better utilization of resources without harming quality may be hard for doctors and patients to accept. Doctors have to be prepared to "kill some sacred cows," in the words of Robert B. Talley, M.D., a gastroenterologist in Stockton, California, and another leader in quality-of-care evaluation.

"Many of us learned in training," said Dr. Talley, "that a gastric-ulcer patient had to be hospitalized for three weeks, put on a strict antacid regimen, and repeatedly X-rayed. If the ulcer wasn't healed in three weeks, you did more tests and wrote down 'cancer of the stomach.' Today, ulcer patients are treated out of the hospital most of the time, with results that are as good or better." Efforts like these to bring about improved quality of care, or the same level of quality, at no additional cost often have side benefits by minimizing the risks of continued hospitalization or extra procedures. Every time a patient stays in the hospital an extra day or two he runs the risk of developing an infection, falling out of bed, or developing a bedsore. Every additional X ray or other diagnostic procedure that isn't absolutely necessary increases to some extent the risk of something going wrong.

It isn't always the doctors who bring the pressure for more time in the hospital or for more diagnostic procedures. Patients do so, too, out of a desire to collect on health insurance—or sometimes out of fear. Warren Nestler, M.D., of Overlook Hospital, describes a study on concussion management in the hospital emergency department. Limited indications for skull X ray had been spelled out, yet doctors were failing to follow the guidelines 53 percent of the time the first year, and 81 percent of the time the following year. "The doctors were ordering far more X rays than were indicated," Dr. Nestler says. Why? Because the mothers said, ". . . but you didn't take an X ray. Aren't you going to?" If the emergency room physician said "No," the mother often said, "I'll find another doctor to X-ray my child's head." So the doctor finds it easier to break a quality standard than to try to convince an upset mother.

With all these gray areas of judgment, I have concluded that it is much easier to identify a really bad doctor or a really bad error in medical care than it is to determine what good-quality care is and how much the care you may receive will vary from that standard. The results of research are always changing the ground rules for doctors. If they have trouble keeping up with the definition of "quality," how can patients expect to know exactly what constitutes good quality care?

But, on the positive side, I have found that the medical profession in the United States is farther ahead in trying to assess quality and to improve it than are health-care systems in most other countries of the world. If doctors, hospitals, and the public at large continue to work on improving the available resources for care, if they continue to set standards for the processes of care and continue to look hard at the outcome, including the patient satisfaction, then the overall quality of care should continue to improve.

And if you and I take the responsibility for our own health and health care, we'll be in the best position possible to take advantage of the best care available to us and our families.

HEALTH HISTORY QUESTIONNAIRE *

The health history questionnaire on the following pages is important to you and your doctor. It gives him information he needs about your health that only you can tell him. When it is completed, take it with you on your next appointment. The questionnaire is divided into sections. Please read the instructions given with each section before answering the questions. Please PRINT when you are asked to complete information. Make an (X) where you are asked to do so.

Do not worry about questions you cannot answer. If you are not sure how a question should be answered, place a solid circle (●) in the "Yes" column or in the space provided if it is not a "Yes/No" question. You will have a chance to go over these questions with the doctor during your appointment.

IDENTIFICATION DATA   Please print the following information.

File no. _____

Date _____

Name _____

Date of birth _____   — Male   — Female

Address _____

— Married — Separated — Divorced — Widowed — Single

Education: — years Elementary — years High School

— years College, Technical, Business, etc.

Home telephone _____
(area code)

Occupation _____

Business telephone _____
(area code)

FAMILY HISTORY:
For each family member below, follow the line across the page and mark an X in those boxes which indicate their present state of health (good), (poor), or their death (write in the cause), and any of the illnesses that they have ever had.

If married, print the names of your spouse and children in the spaces below.

| | Health | | | Cause of death | Allergies or asthma | Anemia | Bleed easily | Diabetes | Cancer or tumor | Epilepsy | Glaucoma | Genetic disease | Alcoholism | Kidney or bladder trouble | Stomach / duodenal ulcer | Nervous breakdown | Rheumatism or arthritis | High blood pressure | Heart trouble | Gout |
	Good	Poor	Died																	
Father:																				
Mother:																				
Brothers or Sisters:																				
Spouse:																				
Child:																				
Child:																				
Child:																				
Child:																				
Child:																				
Paternal relatives (write how many affected in each box) →																				
Maternal relatives (write how many affected in each box) →																				

YOUR HEALTH HISTORY (begin here with illnesses) ——→

Additional Illnesses or Problems: Mark an X in the box next to any of the following that you have now or have ever had.

- ☐ eye infections
- ☐ thyroid disease
- ☐ eczema
- ☐ hives or rashes
- ☐ bronchitis
- ☐ emphysema

- ☐ pneumonia
- ☐ pancreatitis
- ☐ liver disease
- ☐ diverticulosis
- ☐ hernia
- ☐ hemorrhoids

- ☐ neuralgia or neuritis
- ☐ tension/anxiety
- ☐ depression
- ☐ childhood hyperactivity
- ☐ chicken pox
- ☐ German measles

- ☐ scarlet fever
- ☐ measles
- ☐ mumps
- ☐ polio
- ☐ rheumatic fever
- ☐ malaria

- ☐ mononucleosis
- ☐ venereal disease
- ☐ yellow jaundice
- ☐ other
- ☐
- ☐

Have you ever been turned down for life insurance, military service or employment because of health problems? .... _____ Yes _____ No

Major Hospitalizations: If you have ever been hospitalized for any serious medical illness or operation, write in your most recent hospitalizations below. Check this box ☐ if you have had more than three such hospitalizations. (Do not include normal pregnancies)

	Year	Operation or Illness	Name of Hospital	City and State
1st hospitalization				
2nd hospitalization				
3rd hospitalization				

Tests and Immunizations: Mark an X next to those that you have had. Enter the year when you last were given the test or "shots."

Year		Year	
☐ 19___ chest x-ray		☐ 19___ smallpox "shots"	
☐ 19___ kidney x-ray		☐ 19___ tetanus "shots"	
☐ 19___ G.I. series		☐ 19___ polio series	
☐ 19___ colon x-ray		☐ 19___ typhoid "shots"	
☐ 19___ gallbladder x-ray		☐ 19___ flu injections	
☐ 19___ electrocardiogram		☐ 19___ mumps "shots"	
☐ 19___ TB test		☐ 19___ measles "shots"	
☐ 19___ other x-rays		☐ 19___ other	

Medicines: Mark an X in the box next to any medicines that you are now taking, or that you are sensitive or allergic to:

	allergic			allergic	
taking	to:		taking	to:	
☐	☐	antibiotics	☐	☐	aspirin
☐	☐	penicillin	☐	☐	diet pills
☐	☐	sulfa	☐	☐	antacids
☐	☐	opiates/codeine	☐	☐	laxatives
☐	☐	diuretics/water pills	☐	☐	cold tablets
☐	☐	sedatives	☐	☐	_____
☐	☐	stimulants/caffeine	☐	☐	_____
☐	☐	Demerol	☐	☐	
☐	☐	blood pressure medicine			

CONTINUE TO NEXT PAGE

Signature (if filled out by other than patient): _____

Please answer each of the following questions by placing an (X) in the "Yes" blank at the right if your answer to the question is yes, or by placing an (X) in the "No" blank at the right if your answer to the question is no. If you are unable to answer for any reason, place a solid circle (●) in the "Yes" blank.

1. Are you troubled with stiff or painful muscles or joints? .... 1. ____ Yes ____ No
2. Are your joints ever swollen? .... 2. ____ Yes ____ No
3. Are you troubled by pains in the back or shoulder? .... 3. ____ Yes ____ No
4. Are your feet often painful? .... 4. ____ Yes ____ No
5. Are you handicapped in any way? .... 5. ____ Yes ____ No

6. Do you have any skin problems? .... 6. ____ Yes ____ No
7. Does your skin itch or burn? .... 7. ____ Yes ____ No
8. Do you have trouble stopping even a small cut from bleeding? ..... 8. ____ Yes ____ No
9. Do you bruise easily? .... 9. ____ Yes ____ No

10. Do you ever faint or feel faint? .... 10. ____ Yes ____ No
11. Is any part of your body always numb? .... 11. ____ Yes ____ No
12. Have you ever had fits or convulsions? .... 12. ____ Yes ____ No
13. Has your handwriting changed lately? .... 13. ____ Yes ____ No
14. Do you have a tendency to shake or tremble? .... 14. ____ Yes ____ No

15. Are you very nervous around strangers? .... 15. ____ Yes ____ No
16. Do you find it hard to make decisions? .... 16. ____ Yes ____ No
17. Do you find it hard to concentrate or remember? .... 17. ____ Yes ____ No
18. Do you usually feel lonely or depressed? .... 18. ____ Yes ____ No
19. Do you often cry? .... 19. ____ Yes ____ No
20. Would you say you have a hopeless outlook? .... 20. ____ Yes ____ No
21. Do you have difficulty relaxing? .... 21. ____ Yes ____ No
22. Do you have a tendency to worry a lot? .... 22. ____ Yes ____ No
23. Are you troubled by frightening dreams or thoughts? .... 23. ____ Yes ____ No
24. Do you have a tendency to be shy or sensitive? .... 24. ____ Yes ____ No
25. Do you have a strong dislike for criticism? .... 25. ____ Yes ____ No
26. Do you lose your temper often? .... 26. ____ Yes ____ No
27. Do little things often annoy you? .... 27. ____ Yes ____ No
28. Are you disturbed by any work or family problems? .... 28. ____ Yes ____ No
29. Are you having any sexual difficulties? .... 29. ____ Yes ____ No
30. Have you ever considered committing suicide? .... 30. ____ Yes ____ No
31. Have you ever desired or sought psychiatric help? .... 31. ____ Yes ____ No

32. Have you gained or lost much weight recently? .... 32. ____ Yes ____ No
33. Do you have a tendency to be too hot or too cold? .... 33. ____ Yes ____ No
34. Have you lost your interest in eating lately? .... 34. ____ Yes ____ No

35. Do you always seem to be hungry?..................... 35. ____ Yes ____ No
36. Are you more thirsty than usual lately?................. 36. ____ Yes ____ No
37. Are there any swellings in your armpits or groin? .... 37. ____ Yes ____ No
38. Do you seem to feel exhausted or fatigued most of the time? ... 38. ____ Yes ____ No
39. Do you have difficulty either falling asleep or staying asleep? .. 39. ____ Yes ____ No
40. Do you fail to get the exercise you should?............... 40. ____ Yes ____ No
41. Do you smoke?.................................... 41. ____ Yes ____ No
42. Do you take two or more alcoholic drinks a day?........... 42. ____ Yes ____ No
43. Do you drink more than six cups of coffee or tea a day?...... 43. ____ Yes ____ No
44. Have you ever used marijuana? .... 44. ____ Yes ____ No
45. Have you ever used heroin, LSD, or similar drugs?.......... 45. ____ Yes ____ No
46. Do you bite your nails?............................. 46. ____ Yes ____ No
47. Do you often ride in cars without using any safety belts?...... 47. ____ Yes ____ No
48. List any country outside the United States you have visited in
    the past six months .... 48. _____
49. Are you troubled by heartburn? .... 49. ____ Yes ____ No
50. Do you feel bloated after eating? .... 50. ____ Yes ____ No
51. Are you troubled by belching? .... 51. ____ Yes ____ No
52. Do you suffer discomfort in the pit of your stomach?........ 52. ____ Yes ____ No
53. Do you easily become nauseated (feel like vomiting)?........ 53. ____ Yes ____ No
54. Have you ever vomited blood?........................ 54. ____ Yes ____ No
55. Is it difficult or painful for you to swallow? .... 55. ____ Yes ____ No
56. Are you constipated more than twice a month? .... 56. ____ Yes ____ No
57. Are your bowel movements ever loose for more than one day? .. 57. ____ Yes ____ No
58. Are your bowel movements ever black or bloody? .... 58. ____ Yes ____ No
59. Are your bowel movements ever grey in color? .... 59. ____ Yes ____ No
60. Do you suffer pains when you move your bowels?........... 60. ____ Yes ____ No
61. Have you had any bleeding from your rectum? .... 61. ____ Yes ____ No

62. Do you frequently get up at night to urinate? .... 62. ____ Yes ____ No
63. Do you urinate more than five or six times a day? .... 63. ____ Yes ____ No
64. Do you wet your pants or wet your bed?................. 64. ____ Yes ____ No
65. Have you ever had burning or pains when you urinate?....... 65. ____ Yes ____ No
66. Has your urine ever been brown, black or bloody? .... 66. ____ Yes ____ No
67. Do you have any difficulty starting your urine flow? .... 67. ____ Yes ____ No
68. Do you have a constant feeling that you have to urinate?...... 68. ____ Yes ____ No

For Men Only

69. Is your urine stream very weak and slow? .... 69. ____ Yes ____ No
70. Has a doctor ever told you that you have prostate trouble? .... 70. ____ Yes ____ No
71. Have you had any burning or discharge from your penis? ..... 71. ____ Yes ____ No
72. Are there any swellings or lumps on your testicles?.......... 72. ____ Yes ____ No
73. Do your testicles get painful? .... 73. ____ Yes ____ No

For Women Only

74. Are you having trouble with your menstrual periods?..........74. ____ Yes ____ No
75. Have you ever had bleeding between your periods?..........75. ____ Yes ____ No
76. Do you have heavy bleeding with your periods?..............76. ____ Yes ____ No
77. Do you ever have bleeding after intercourse? ....77. ____ Yes ____ No
78. Do you feel bloated and irritable before your period? ....78. ____ Yes ____ No
79. Do you have hot flashes?.............................79. ____ Yes ____ No
80. Have you ever taken any birth control pills?.................80. ____ Yes ____ No
81. Have you ever had any lumps in your breasts?..............81. ____ Yes ____ No
82. Have you had any excessive discharges from your vagina?......82. ____ Yes ____ No
83. Please print the month and year of your last PAP smear.......83. _____
84. Please print the date your last menstrual period began........84. _____
Print the following information in the spaces at the right:
85. Number of pregnancies..............................85. _____
86. Number of miscarriages ....86. _____
87. Number of stillbirths ....87. _____
88. Number of premature births ....88. _____
89. Number of children born alive.........................89. _____
90. Number of cesarean operations ....90. _____
91. Have you ever had an abortion?........................91. ____ Yes ____ No

92. Do you have headaches more than once a week?.............92. ____ Yes ____ No
93. Does twisting your neck quickly cause pain?................93. ____ Yes ____ No
94. Have you ever had lumps or swelling in your neck?..........94. ____ Yes ____ No

95. Do you wear glasses? ....95. ____ Yes ____ No
96. Does your eyesight ever blur? ....96. ____ Yes ____ No
97. Is your eyesight getting worse?.........................97. ____ Yes ____ No
98. Do you ever see double? ....98. ____ Yes ____ No
99. Do you ever see colored halos around lights? ....99. ____ Yes ____ No
100. Do you ever have pains or itching in or around your eyes? ....100. ____ Yes ____ No
101. Do your eyes blink or water most of the time?..............101. ____ Yes ____ No
102. Have you had any trouble with your eyes in the last two years? .102. ____ Yes ____ No

103. Do you have difficulty hearing? ....103. ____ Yes ____ No
104. Have you had any earaches lately?......................104. ____ Yes ____ No
105. Have you been troubled by running ears lately?.............105. ____ Yes ____ No
106. Do you have a repeated buzzing or other noises in your ears? ..106. ____ Yes ____ No
107. Do you get motion sickness riding in a car or plane?.........107. ____ Yes ____ No

108. Do you have any problems with your teeth?................108. ____ Yes ____ No

109. Do you have any sore swellings on your gums or jaws? . . . . . . .109. _____ Yes _____ No
110. Is your tongue sore or sensitive? . . . . .110. _____ Yes _____ No
111. Have your taste senses changed lately? . . . . .111. _____ Yes _____ No

112. Is your nose stuffed up when you don't have a cold? . . . . .112. _____ Yes _____ No
113. Does your nose run when you don't have a cold? . . . . .113. _____ Yes _____ No
114. Do you ever have sneezing spells? . . . . .114. _____ Yes _____ No
115. Do you ever have head colds two or more months in a row? . . . .115. _____ Yes _____ No
116. Does your nose ever bleed for no reason at all? . . . . .116. _____ Yes _____ No
117. Is your throat ever sore when you don't have a cold? . . . . .117. _____ Yes _____ No
118. Has a doctor told you that your tonsils have been enlarged? . . . .118. _____ Yes _____ No
119. Has your voice ever been hoarse when you didn't have a cold? .119. _____ Yes _____ No

120. Do you wheeze or have to gasp to breathe? . . . . .120. _____ Yes _____ No
121. Are you bothered by coughing spells? .121. _____ Yes _____ No
122. Do you cough up a lot of phlegm (thick spit)? . . . . .122. _____ Yes _____ No
123. Have you ever coughed up blood? . . . . .123. _____ Yes _____ No
124. Do you get chest colds more than once a month? . . . . .124. _____ Yes _____ No
125. Are you sweating more than usual or having night sweats? . . . . .125. _____ Yes _____ No

126. Have you ever been told that you had high blood pressure? . . . .126. _____ Yes _____ No
127. Have you been bothered by a thumping or racing heart? . . . . . .127. _____ Yes _____ No
128. Do you ever get pains or tightness in your chest? . . . . .128. _____ Yes _____ No
129. Do you have trouble with dizziness or lightheadedness? . . . . . . .129. _____ Yes _____ No
130. Does every little effort leave you short of breath? . . . . .130. _____ Yes _____ No
131. Do you wake up at night short of breath? . . . . .131. _____ Yes _____ No
132. Are you using more pillows to help you breathe at night? . . . . . .132. _____ Yes _____ No
133. Do you have trouble with swollen feet or ankles? . . . . .133. _____ Yes _____ No
134. Are you getting cramps in your legs at night or upon walking? . .134. _____ Yes _____ No
135. Have you ever been told that you have a heart murmur? . . . . . .135. _____ Yes _____ No

Now, in the blank lines below please describe any special problems or symptoms that you wish to discuss with the doctor.

_____

_____

_____

_____

PERSONAL HEALTH PROFILE *

Carry this with you at all times.

Review with your physician at each visit.

WARNING!

I (am) (have) _____

Identification Data:

Name _____

Address _____

City _____ State _____ Zip_____

Home Tel. _____

Health Ins. Co and No. _____

In emergency, please notify:

Name _____ Tel. _____

Physician _____ Tel. _____

Prob. No.	Significant Problems	Status		Prob. No.	Medications	Dosage	Dates	
		A	R				Start	Stop

A=Active   R=Resolved

Sensitivities
to medication

Blood Type: Vision Rx:

PERSONAL HEALTH PROFILE *

Carry this with you at all times.

Review with your physician at each visit.

WARNING!

I (am) (have) _____

Identification Data:

Name _____

Address _____

City _____ State _____ Zip_____

Home Tel. _____

Health Ins. Co and No. _____

In emergency, please notify:

Name _____ Tel. _____

Physician _____ Tel. _____

Prob. No.	Significant Problems	Status A	Status R	Prob. No.	Medications	Dosage	Dates Start	Dates Stop

A=Active   R=Resolved

Sensitivities
to medication

Blood Type: Vision Rx:

PERSONAL HEALTH PROFILE *

Carry this with you at all times.

Review with your physician at each visit.

WARNING!

I (am) (have) _____

Identification Data:

Name _____

Address _____

City _____ State _____ Zip_____

Home Tel. _____

Health Ins. Co and No. _____

In emergency, please notify:

Name _____ Tel. _____

Physician _____ Tel. _____

Prob. No.	Significant Problems	Status A	Status R	Prob. No.	Medications	Dosage	Dates Start	Stop

A=Active   R=Resolved

	Sensitivities to medication

Blood Type: Vision Rx:

PERSONAL HEALTH PROFILE *

Carry this with you at all times.
Review with your physician at each visit.

WARNING!

I (am) (have) _____

Identification Data:

Name _____

Address _____

City _____ State _____ Zip_____

Home Tel. _____

Health Ins. Co and No. _____

In emergency, please notify:

Name _____ Tel. _____

Physician _____ Tel. _____

Prob. No.	Significant Problems	Status A	Status R	Prob. No.	Medications	Dosage	Dates Start	Dates Stop

A=Active   R=Resolved

Sensitivities
to medication

Blood Type: Vision Rx:

• © 1978 Miller Communications, Inc.

PERSONAL HEALTH PROFILE*
Carry this with you at all times.
Review with your physician at each visit.

WARNING!

I (am) (have) _____

Identification Data:

Name _____

Address _____

City _____ State _____ Zip_____

Home Tel. _____

Health Ins. Co and No. _____

In emergency, please notify:

Name _____ Tel. _____

Physician _____ Tel. _____

Prob. No.	Significant Problems	Status A	Status R	Prob. No.	Medications	Dosage	Dates Start	Stop

A=Active   R=Resolved

Sensitivities to medication

Blood Type: Vision Rx:

PERSONAL HEALTH PROFILE *

Carry this with you at all times.

Review with your physician at each visit.

WARNING!

I (am) (have) _____

Identification Data:

Name _____

Address _____

City _____ State _____ Zip_____

Home Tel. _____

Health Ins. Co and No. _____

In emergency, please notify:

Name _____ Tel. _____

Physician _____ Tel. _____

Prob. No.	Significant Problems	Status A	Status R	Prob. No.	Medications	Dosage	Dates Start	Dates Stop

A=Active   R=Resolved

Sensitivities
to medication

Blood Type: Vision Rx:

INDEX

This Index has been prepared as a supplement to the Contents. If you are unable to find a listing here, please consult the subheadings in the Contents.

Accreditation
  manual on, 159
  of hospitals, Joint Commission on, 165–166, 172, 183, 254–255
  of nursing homes, 194–195
Aging, Office of
  for information on residential-care facilities, 185
  See also Nursing homes
Alcoholism
  seeking your physician's advice on, 105–106
Allergy
  as a specialty, 40
Allied health professionals
  and house calls, 126
  physician extenders, 51–54
  See also Nursing
Alvarez, Walter C., 24

American Board of Family Practice, 253–254
American Cancer Society, 109
American Hospital Association and Patient's Bill of Rights, 178–180
American Medical Association
  and physician education, 37
  and recommendation on physicians' fees, 228
  attitude toward chiropractic, 50
  attitude toward osteopathy, 50
  principles of medical ethics, 137
  Professional Recognition Award, 37

American Nursing Home Association, 246
American Osteopathic Association, 47
American Society of Internal Medicine, 145–146
Anonsen, Richard E., 255
Anxiety
  See Emotional problems

Berry, Ralph, 160
Blue Cross and Blue Shield
  individuals vs. group coverage, 209
  seeking advice on, 210
  service benefits, 205
  supplemental insurance for Medicare, 219
  surgical consultation, 161
Bowel problems
  possible causes of, 81

California Medical Association, 226
Cancer treatment centers, 108, 166
Cardiology
  See Heart disease
Carmichael, Lynn, 97–98
Checklists
  See Patient guidelines
Checkups, periodic
  clinics for, 65–66
  for adults, 62, 63–64
  for adults, types of tests included, 67–69
  for children, 60–62
  for children, preventive care plan, 69ff.
  for older people, 64–65
  physician opinions on, 57–60
  reasons for having, 62–63, 67
Children
  checkups, guidelines for, 60–62, 65
  family physician and, 30, 40–41
  patient checklist of topics to discuss with physician, 106
  pediatrics, as a specialty, 42
  pediatrics, combined with internal medicine, for family care, 31
  preventive care plan for, 69ff.
Chiropody
  See Podiatry
Chiropractic, 50
Clinics
  for periodic checkups, 65–66
  group practices, 30, 32
  using Health Hazard Appraisal, where to write for list of, 60
Commission on Professional and Hospital Activities, 160
Committee on Education in Family Life
  checklist of topics to discuss with your physician, 106
Costs
  of drugs, comparison shopping, 247
  of hospitals, 232–234
  of hospitals, how to control, 242–245

of hospitals, monitoring of, 235
of hospitals, physician familiarity with, 234
of nursing homes, 195–196, 235–236
of nursing homes, how to control, 243–244, 245–246
of periodic checkups, 66–67
of physicians, 246–248
of private duty nursing, 243–244
of tests, 248
patient checklist of topics to discuss with the physician, 106
what to do about overcharging, 239–240

Dental problems
dentists and, 49
guidelines for choosing dentists, 33–35
infections following therapy for, 87–88
insurance coverage for, 204
Dermatology
as a specialty, 44
Diabetes
patient attitudes on, 92–94
Dizziness
possible causes of, 77
Drugs
insurance coverage of, 203
obtaining information on, 95–96
physician attitude toward, 133–134
price comparisons of, 247

reactions to, recording in Personal Health Profile, 115–116, 265–273

Ears
hearing trouble, possible causes of, 78
otolaryngology, as a specialty, 44
Eating
problems associated with, 75–76
Eiseman, Ben, 242
Emergencies
as reason for office delays, 120
chest pain, 79
deciding on what constitutes an emergency, 75
emergency rooms, 30, 112–113, 127–128, 248
heart attacks, 71–72
house calls, 125–126
nausea and vomiting, 76
physician responsibility in, 149–150
Emergency rooms
See Emergencies
Emery, Lydia, 221
Emotional problems
alcoholism, 105–106
emotional impact of surgery, 162
family crises, 103–104
marital conflicts, 103
patient checklist of topics to discuss with physician, 106
possible causes of, 78

Emotional problems (*cont.*)
sexual problems, how to discuss them with the physician, 102–103
sexual problems, possible causes of, 80
See also Psychiatry; Psychology
Eyes
ophthalmology, as a specialty, 44
problems of, 77

Family care
advice on residential care facilities, 185
alcoholism, 105–106
as a specialty, 40–41
checklist of topics to discuss with your physician, 106
checkups and, 65
family conference on nursing homes, 190–191
family physician, schedule of, 126–127
family problems, 103–104
from different specialties, 30
marital conflicts, 103
sexual problems, 80, 102–103
See also Children
Family practice
as a specialty, 40–41
See also Family care; Primary care
Fatigue
possible causes of, 77

Federal health insurance
monitoring of, by Professional Standards Review Organizations, 172–173
See also Medicaid; Medicare
Friedman, W. R., Jr., 234

Gastroenterology
as a specialty, 42
General practitioners
for primary family care, 30
See also Family care; Family practice
Gibbs, Richard F., 159, 162
Green, Lawrence W., 92
Group practice
See Clinics

Hackett, Thomas P., 72
Harper, C. Wallace, 224–225
Health examinations
See Checkups, periodic
Health Hazard Appraisal
importance of environmental medical history in, 89–90
where to write for list of clinics using, 60
Health History Questionnaire, 258–264
Health Insurance Association of America, 210
Health maintenance organizations (HMOs), 208–209
and physicians' fees, 222
Health Systems Agencies, 249

Heart disease
and warning about infections following dental work, 87–88
cardiology, as a specialty, 41–42
heart attacks, when to seek help for, 71–72
patients with, and memory of presurgery discussion, 163
Herman, Lawrence, 71
Hoff, David L., 59
Hospice programs, 110–111
Hospital privileges
and your physician, 38–39, 164, 169–170
hospital quality restrictions, 254
role of credentials committee, 173
Hospitals
accreditation for, by Joint Commission on Accreditation of Hospitals, 165–166, 172, 183, 254–255
charges of, 232–234
Council on Teaching Hospitals, 167
how to control costs of stay in, 242–245
insurance coverage for stay in, 203
monitoring of costs in, 235
Patient's Bill of Rights, 178–180
standards for physicians practicing in, 254
See also Hospital privileges; Malpractice

Huffman, B. Leslie, 57
Hunt, Vincent R., 57–58

Insomnia
possible causes of, 77
Institute of Medicine, National Academy of Sciences, 250–251
Internal medicine
as a specialty, 41
for primary care, 30
subspecialties of, 41–42

Joint Commission on Accreditation of Hospitals, 165–166, 172, 183, 254–255
Journal of Legal Medicine, 159

Lafferty, Wayne, 121–122
Lane, Walter, 121–122
Leaman, Thomas L., 100
"Living Will," 99
Lohrenz, Francis N., 57, 58

Malpractice
American Society of Internal Medicine statement on, 145–146
defining competence, 145
hospital credentials committee, 173
hospital overcharging, 239–240
hospital quality restrictions, 254

Malpractice (*cont.*)
Medicaid abuses, 219
Patient's Bill of Rights, 178–180
physician overcharging, 238–239
physician responsibility in emergencies and, 149–150
seeking other opinions, 138–141, 161
standards for lawsuits, 146–148
study on patient dissatisfaction, 144
Manning, Robert, 57
Massachusetts General Hospital, 155–156
Maternity benefits
under maternal/child federal health insurance, 203
Mayo Clinic, 24, 58, 82
M. D. Anderson Hospital and Tumor Institute (University of Texas), 108, 166
Medicaid
benefits of, 216–217
definition of, 215–216
monitoring of by Professional Standards Review Organizations, 172–173
state costs of, 242
Medical Economics magazine, 22, 120, 221–222, 240
Medical education
See Professional qualifications
Medical Records
and emergency rooms, 248
keeping a record of injections, 95

Personal Health Profile, 114–117
reviewing examination reports, 66
transfer of, 113–114
Medicare
"Assignment," 218, 219
benefits of, 216
definition of, 215–216
monitoring of, by Professional Standards Review Organizations, 172–173
"Your Medicare Handbook," 220
Memorial Hospital–Sloane-Kettering Institute for Cancer Research, 108, 166
Menstrual problems
patient checklist of topics to discuss with your physician, 106
possible causes of, 78
Millikan, Clark, 82
Millis, John H., 30
Minnesota State Medical Association, 151

National Academy of Sciences Institute of Medicine, 250–251
National Ambulatory Medical Care Survey, 70, 72
National Cancer Institute, 109
National Jewish Hospital, 166
Nestler, Warren, 257
Nose problems
See Otolaryngology
Nursing
coordination of, 174

costs of, 243–244
insurance coverage of, 204
nurse practitioners, independent, 53–54
nursing home care, 191
patient advocate, 174–175
private-duty nurses, 176
RN's and non-RN's, 175
Nursing homes
checklist for, 197–199
costs of, 195–196, 235–236
cost control, 243–244, 245–246
Office of Aging, for information on residential-care facilities, 185
rehabilitative services in, 246

Obstetrics and gynecology
as a specialty, 42–43
for primary care, 30, 42
maternal/child federal health insurance, monitoring of, 172–173
maternity benefits, 203
patient checklist of topics to discuss with your physician, 106
Ophthalmology
as a specialty, 44
eye problems, 77
Optometry, 49–50
Osteopathy, 46–47
Otolaryngology
as a specialty, 44
Overlook Hospital, 250–251, 252–253, 257

Pain
possible causes of, 79
Palpitations
possible causes of, 77
Patient advocate
in hospital and community, 174–175
Patient Care magazine, 22, 92, 158
Patient guidelines
for family health insurance, 212–213
for nursing homes, 197–199
for periodic checkups, 60–63, 64–65, 67–69
Health History Questionnaire, 258–264
"Living Will," 99
Patient's Bill of Rights, 178–180
Personal Health Profiles, 115–116, 265–273
topics to discuss with your physician, 106
Pathology
as aid to diagnosis and treatment, 44
Pediatrics
as a specialty, 42
checklist of topics to discuss with your physician, 106
checkups for children, 60–62
combined with internal medicine, for family care, 31
preventive care plan, 69ff.
risks of tonsillectomy in children, 160–161
Personal Health Profile, 115–116, 265–273

Podiatry, 48–49
Prevention, disease
  and control of medical costs, 248–249
  by periodic checkups, 57
  minimum plan for preventive care in children, 69ff.
  role of life-style changes in, 58–59
Primary care
  advice on residential-care facilities, 185
  how to choose a physician for, 29–35
  in nursing, 174
  physician and questions about hospitalization, 156
  physician and referrals to consultants, 138
  physician to coordinate care of specialists, 174
Professional qualifications
  for chiropractic, 50
  for dentistry, 49
  for optometry, 49–50
  for osteopathy, 46–47
  for podiatry, 48–49
  for psychology, 47–48
  how to find a physician, 33–35
  physician education, 37
  practical experience, 39
  specialty board certification, 37–38
  See also Hospital privileges; Malpractice
Professional Standards Review Organizations, 172–173, 255
Psychiatry
  as a specialty, 43

emotional impact of surgery, 162
emotional problems, possible causes of, 78
insurance coverage of, 204
Psychology
  emotional impact of surgery, 162
  emotional problems, possible causes of, 78
  psychologists, 47–48

Radiology
  as a specialty, 44–45
Rehabilitation
  day-care centers, 187–188
  home health care, 186–187
  in extended care facilities, 182–183
  in nursing-care facilities, 183–184
  Medicare and Medicaid benefits, 216–217
  See also Nursing homes
Relative value studies
  for physicians' fees, 226–227
Respiratory problems
  possible causes of, 80
Richmond, Virginia Medical Society, 144
Robbins, Lewis C., 60
Robinson, George, 163
Roswell Park Memorial Institute, 108
Roth, Russell B., 234

Sexual problems
  how to discuss with your physician, 102–103

patient checklist, as aid in, 106
possible causes of, 80
Simmons, Henry E., 256
Skin problems
possible causes of, 80–81
Surgery
as a specialty, 43–44
consultation on, and Blue Cross–Blue Shield, 161
coverage of by health insurance, 203
guidelines for physician's hospital visits, 128
heart, ability of patients to remember presurgery discussion, 163
how to control costs of, 243
outpatient surgery departments, 155
risks of tonsillectomy in children, 160–161
seeking other opinions on, 138, 140
Symptoms
importance of, 75–81

See also specific symptoms

Talley, Robert B., 256
Teeling-Smith, George, 70
Tests
costs of, 232, 243, 248
diagnostic, insurance coverage of, 203
included in periodic checkup, 67–69
physician attitude toward, 132–133
Trautlein, Joseph J., 58
Trembling
possible causes of, 77

Urinary problems
possible causes of, 81

Washington State Medical Association, 151
Weakness
possible causes of, 77